WEIGHT LOSS
UNLOCKED

A Total Weight-Loss, Diet, and Fitness Guide

By Paul J.R. Dawson

Freebird Publishers

North Dighton, MA

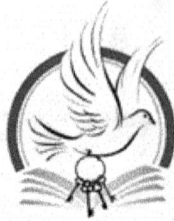

Freebird Publishers
221 Pearl St., Ste. 541, North Dighton, MA 02764
Info@FreebirdPublishers.com
www.FreebirdPublishers.com

Copyright © 2020
Weight Loss Unlocked
A Total Weight-Loss, Diet, and Fitness Guide
By Paul J.R. Dawson

All Freebird Publishers titles, imprints, and distributed lines are available at special quantity discounts for bulk purchases for sales promotions, premiums, fundraising, educational, or institutional use.

ISBN: 978-1-952159-20-6

Printed in the United States of America

DEDICATION

This book is dedicated to every single person who said that this was impossible and couldn't be done. Honestly, thank you! You helped me pull all-nighters, skip TV shows, meals, and work all month to pay for copies and priority envelopes (in other words: no commissary).

Without you, none of this would be possible.

DISCLAIMER

The author of this book is not a physician and is not licensed to give medical advice. The information in this book has been gathered for the convenience of the reader. The information in this book is subject to change and may differ from the original works. The revision done herein was prior to 2022. This information does not constitute a recommendation or endorsement of any individual, product, or institution, nor is it intended as a substitute for individualized consultation with your physician. The author and publisher deny any liability arising directly or indirectly from the use of this book.

This book in no way is a replacement for a well-balanced, nutritional diet. This book is a collection of recipes that the author enjoys and has used to help him lose weight. Results may vary. Be sure to check with a certified physician before changing your diet. Be sure to follow medical professional advice.

All recipes in this book are portioned out for one person. Check with your facility before cooking meals for multiple people.

This book is not intended as a substitute for the medical advice of a physical therapist or physician. If you suspect that you may have any specific medical issues, contact medical professionals immediately regarding any of the recommendations made in this book.

Further, the author and publisher have done their best to ensure that the workouts suggested are safe. However, the author and publisher take no responsibility for any injury, strain, sprain, or any accident resulting from any of the activities mentioned herein. The author and publisher advise you to stay safe and aware.

TABLE OF CONTENTS

Dedication iii

Disclaimer.. iv

Table of Contents 1

PART ONE: Weight Loss Unlocked....................................7

Weight Chart.. 8

Introduction, Part 1 9

About Me and Weight 10

Avocados in Prison?... 11

Goal of this Section.. 12

Chapter One.. 13

Carbohydrate Wean System 13

Enemy List.. 13

Week 1 (7 Days)... 14

Week 2 (7 Days)... 15

Week 3 (7 Days)... 16

Week 4 (7 Days)... 17

Drayvon's Carbohydrate Wean Experience.............................. 18

Carb Wean Tip 19

Chapter Two.. 22

Intermittent Fasting 22

What's Intermittent Fasting? 24

Intermittent Fasting Styles 28

Chapter Three 35

Common Questions & Concerns... 35

Intermittent Whaaa?..38

Chapter Four 40

  Water Works! What You Need To Know About H20 40

    Water and Your Health..40

    Benefits of Water 43

    30-Day H_2O Gallon Challenge 46

    Water Challenge Calendar.....................................48

    Sorry Cellie! 48

Chapter Five 51

  Prisoner's Nutrition Guide 51

    Calories..52

    Fat...55

    Saturated Fat...56

    Cholesterol 57

    Protein 58

    Carbohydrates 60

    Sugar...61

    Fiber...63

    Calcium 64

    Sodium..65

    Potassium 66

    Folic Acid..67

    Vitamin C 68

    Dietary Guideline Basics 69

Chapter Six 73

  How to Read Food Labels 73

    Packaging Terms...74

    Secondary Packaging Terms 75

    No Hormones Added ....**Error! Bookmark not defined.**

Thank You Label! 77

Chapter Seven 79

Vitamin & Mineral Guide 79

Vitamins 79

Minerals 81

PART TWO: Cook Book & Meal Guide............................83

Chapter One: Main Dishes 85

Venezuelan Rice 86

Mack Stack.. 87

Vienna Rice 89

Peppered Rice... 90

Pickled Rice 91

BOB (Ballin' on a Budget) Chicken Bowl.................... 92

Orange Rice 93

Mack Chicken Combo 94

Chicken Fried Rice Bowl... 95

The Dippin' Chicken 96

Lemon Pepper Chicken.. 97

Brunch Burritos... 98

Cheesy Chicken Tacos.. 99

Blazin' Tuna Tacos 100

Speedy Chicken Bowl... 101

Southwest Poultry Wraps....................................... 102

Chili Booms 103

The BOB Boom 104

Tuna Booms 105

Jack Mack Booms.. 106

Sardine Booms... 107

Chili Chicken Sof-Chos (Soft Nachos)...................... 108

Cheesy Chicken Sof-Chos.. 109

BOB Sof-Chos... 110

BOB Spicy Sof-Chos.. 111

Chubby Sof-Chos 112

Seafood Poppers Bowl.. 113

Chickety China Chinese Chicken.................................... 114

BOB – OG 115

Crazy Rich Peanut Bowl 116

Sour Mack.. 117

Lemon Fish Lips 118

Screamin' Vegan... 119

3-Rex... 120

Egg Salad... 121

Loaded Jalapeno Bowl... 122

Far East Tuna 123

Meat Shell Tacos... 124

Tuna Crunch 125

Fruit & Chicken Salad.. 126

Health Bowl 127

Chapter Two: Healthy Drinks.. 128

Funny Juice 129

Dragon Tea 130

Hybrid Caddy 131

Mocha Cappuccino 132

Moo-Tea 133

Chai-T.. 134

Lemon Iced Tea 135

Cinna Milk.. 136

Flavor Fusions 137

Tiger Milk 138

Rush Hour 139

Creamy Cocoa 140

Groovy Smoothies 141

The Flood Gate –For Digestive Movement.................. 142

Soothe Aide 143

The Smack Down 144

Chapter Three: Healthy Sweet Treats........................ 146

No Bake Bowl.. 147

Fruity Oatmeal 148

Cinna Rice 149

PBR (Peanut Butter Raisin) Oatmeal 150

Raisin Sun 151

Honey Roasted Oats 152

Chocolate Banana Pudding...................................... 153

The All Natural.. 154

Sugar-Free Taffy 155

Chapter Four: "Chow Time, Chow Time!" 156

Navigating the Chow Hall 158

Breakfasts 159

Lunches 162

Dinners 165

PART THREE: The Exercise Program.......................... 167

Foreword, Part 3... 170

Not My Favorite Thing.. 171

Getting Started... 172

Chapter One: Stretching 174

Foot & Ankle Stretches... 175

Toe Stretches... 176

Foot Stretches 176

Leg Stretches 178

Hip Stretches 180

Back Stretches 181

Shoulder Stretches 183

Elbow Stretches 184

Wrist/Hand Stretches 184

Neck Stretches 185

Yoga Stretches 186

Chapter Two: Exercises 189

Calories Burned by Exercise 190

The 30 Day Walk/Jog Challenge 191

Low Impact Circuit Body Weight Exercises 192

Medium Impact 196

High/Intense Impact Circuit 199

Appendix: 222

DOC Fat and Calorie Guide 222

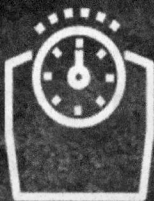

PART 1:
Weight Loss Unlocked

Weight Chart

Height	Weight (Men)	Weight (Women)
5'0"	95-125	90-120
5'1"	105-128	95-120
5'2"	107-133	99-124
5'3"	115-140	105-130
5'4"	118-145	110-135
5'5"	123-152	114-139
5'6"	130-160	118-144
5'7"	135-164	124-150
5'8"	140-171	129-156
5'9"	145-181	132-162
5'10"	152-185	137-169
5'11"	158-191	142-174
6'0"	160-199	145-180
6'1"	165-204	149-185
6'2"	170-210	155-191
6'3"	175-215	159-197

Introduction, Part 1

Welcome! I take it as a great honor that you have decided to give this book a chance. I would like to say thank you! I also take it that since you have this book in your hands, you have been trying all sorts of diets and restrictions, which just don't seem to be working for you. It can be very discouraging to try and fail, maybe ending up worse than when you began. Trust me, I've tried almost all diets available to inmates and lost the weight only to gain even more back.

Luckily, all of those trials and tribulations can be used for good! By going through all of my personal experience and working with over 115 inmates and staff, both male and female, over the course of 10 1/2 years, you can believe that all common denominators have been exposed. This program works for anyone of any age and any gender. People from Eddie C., who looks like he should be playing professional football if it were not for prison, to Officer Walker, who looks like Santa, have been helped by this program (including myself and everyone in between) to lose the weight they wanted and keep it off for years!

The United States is a carbohydrate, sugar-driven country. The prisons of the U.S.A. put that statement on steroids. Every day is a steady stream of bread, potatoes, noodles, rice, beans, cake, pudding, and so many other carbohydrate and sugary products. Let's not even get started on the prison store (commissary, canteen). It's a junk food lover's paradise with a few apparent healthy items. This book will cover some options. Due to this unhealthy environment with little to no options to unlock weight loss results, we need a tool to help us navigate this treacherous terrain. That tool is this book.

Even if you are not incarcerated, you can use the information in here to lose weight. This program is the best thing I've ever done with my life because it helps others.

Bear down, lock in, and get it done! No luck is required! You got this!

About Me and Weight

My name is Paul Dawson. I am not a dietitian or weight loss expert of any kind. I am simply a person who went through a battle with food for more than a decade in prison. I feel that it would be greedy to hoard the information from people who are going through the same battle.

I never really struggled with my weight while I was in the "free world" (not in prison), but then again, I was always on the go and living a very fast life. When I received nearly a life sentence from the judge, I began to eat my pain away. I didn't exercise, I didn't stretch, I just ate and ate and ate. I went from 185 pounds to 260 pounds in a six-month period, 75 pounds!

I eventually worked my way to the Intensive Management Unit (IMU), which some might know as SHU or IDU. Basically, I was not being a good inmate, so I spent 13 months in solitary confinement. Between the exercise I did in the unit and the prison serving smaller portions to IMU inmates, by the time I was released back into the General Population (GP), I weighed 276 pounds. I was very proud of myself. What I failed to realize was that back in GP were all of the products I had been denied for over a year! I could put cocoa in my coffee, eat a bag of nacho cheese chips, large portions in the cafeteria, and so much more. All of these things were horrible for me. Although I continued to exercise, the weight was creeping back.

Sadly, my mother passed away, and I fell into a deep depression. With that, I began eating more and exercising less; eventually, I quit exercising altogether. I was soon up to 268 pounds. A friend named Blue helped me out of this funk, and by running twice a day, I went down to 230 pounds. It was a great start on my path back to 185 pounds, and I had it all figured out. I was 27 then. I can't exactly explain what happened during that last go-round, but when I saw the scale, it was all the motivation I needed.

I am now at 210 pounds and continue to stay down! I feel great and look good. You will feel the same as long as you follow the program. I can't wait to tell you all about it.

Avocados in Prison?

At my heaviest of 276 pounds, I was bound and determined to figure this weight loss thing out. You couldn't believe how excited I was when I saw the commercial for one of the TV doctor shows, which said, "Wednesday, see how this couple lost 400 pounds combined! Tune in, and we'll share their secrets so you can do it too!" I saw this promo on Friday, so I had to wait five days to get the answer. I couldn't wait!

Wednesday came, and I was ready to go at 4 p.m. The show started, and the doctor said, "Welcome. Today, we're going to show you how this husband and wife used avocados, kale, and quinoa to lose over 400 pounds together." My heart sank. Why did it have to be all the things we couldn't get in prison? I tried to stick it out and see if there might be some substitute I could use, but it's almost as if they were expecting someone to be watching and looking for trades and substitutions, because this doctor and this couple were not budging on the benefits of avocado, kale, and quinoa.

That was the day that I decided to write this book. The only roadblock was that I didn't have the right system. After years of trial and error, I finally struck gold and after sharing this program with others and seeing their results. This even includes one correctional officer who lost so much weight and got so healthy that he went to the doctor one day and was told he was no longer diabetic. I knew I had to share this program with the world!

A lot of television programs and magazine articles focus on really expensive and exclusive eating programs that have little to no relevance to the nearly 3,000,000 individuals who are incarcerated in the United States, as well as lower-income Americans who can't afford a majority of the recipes and programs offered by major companies. This book is for *you* and your life because your life is different, and you deserve the information. Don't give up just because you don't get avocados in prison. You can do anything you put your mind to!

Goal of this Section

Although I am bound to say that nothing is guaranteed and all results will vary, the goal that this book intends to accomplish is to teach you about your body and how it processes food, once you understand that your body is burning through certain foods and is storing other foods as fat, you can begin to add or eliminate certain foods from your day-to-day eating schedule. In doing so, you can optimize the burn and eliminate the fat storage, eventually leading your body to burn your fat storage!

I am fully aware that most people with weight issues have spent lots of hours doing research and trying different methods to lose weight. Being overweight doesn't mean we don't know, as a matter of opinion, I believe that overweight people are much more well-read on the topic than others.

With that said, this book is meant for the absolute beginner all the way up to the avid guru. Do not feel insulted if areas of this book are redundant as to what you already know. A lot of time has been spent to make sure all bases of the program are covered, and these methods stick with the reader.

There is not a one-size-fits-all attitude in this book. Once you learn the blueprint, it is best that you adjust it to your needs and your liking. Most importantly, while reading, I want you to laugh, learn, practice, and grow (well, shrink). Have fun, keep a positive mental attitude, and stay focused.

CHAPTER ONE

Carbohydrate Wean System

Enemy List

- Bread
- Potatoes
- Noodles/Pasta
- Chips
- White rice
- Desserts
- Sugary juice
- Soda

Fueling your body is where it all starts. Let's face it, your body is a machine, and it needs fuel to operate. While searching for fuel, carbohydrates are the body's first choice when available. The truth is, carbohydrates are a great source of energy and typically provide that full feeling or satisfied feeling.

We see that there are a lot of prisons and institutions that use carbohydrate-heavy foods on their usual food schedule. Bread, potatoes, noodles/pastas, chips, white rice, desserts, as well as sugary juices and sodas are an inmate's only choice during the course of the day. The problem with this is that once your body has used up the exact amount of carbohydrates needed to give you physical and mental energy for the day, the remaining amount *will* be stored as fat. Your body is a fan of these carbohydrates and doesn't want to lose them, so it hoards them for later. Your body does not care that you already have pounds upon pounds of fat stored from previous excess carbohydrates; it wants more.

Let's say at breakfast, you eat four pancakes, a carbohydrate-heavy food. One of these pancakes has enough grams of carbohydrates to give you energy for the entire day. Your body will break down the other three pancakes into sugar and then store them as fat. Also, any other carbohydrates you consume for the rest of the day will also be broken down and stored as fat.

The proper way to avoid this dilemma is to consume the one pancake in the morning and then do everything in your power to abstain from carbohydrates for the rest of the day. This is going to be helpful in your weight loss journey because by only giving your body enough carbohydrates to put toward energy, it will have nothing to store as fat. Pretty soon, when your body needs energy, it will have no choice but to dig into your fat storage and start burning that stored fat as fuel.

First things first, we need to formulate a plan to wean you from your currently high intake of carbohydrates. Do this as a step-down program, not a cold-turkey approach. You have used massive amounts of carbohydrates for years to power your body and mind. Slowly, you will change your fuel source, but the key word is *slowly*. Following is your plan.

Week 1 (7 Days)

Cut your carbohydrate intake in half; limit desserts to one a week. You know what your preferences are at each meal. At breakfast, if you usually take four slices of toast, take two instead. Take half of the amount of potatoes that you normally get. At lunch, only eat half of the bread; even for a sandwich, just use 1 piece of bread. At dinner, eat half of the spaghetti noodles. Remember, half of the amount of your usual carbohydrate intake is the key. A favorite of mine was pizza night. Keeping in mind the pizza crust (bread) contains the highest amount of carbohydrates, by slicing the pizza in half, taking the toppings off of one half, and putting it all on the other half, I could still enjoy my pizza but with only half of the carbohydrates. Pick one day to eat dessert, *only one*.

If your facility is fortunate enough to provide you with a weekly menu, find out what the meals are so you can plan accordingly. This can be one of your greatest tools as you begin to change your carbohydrate intake. Mentally preparing for the battle that lies ahead is a major step towards winning it. Keep it at the forefront of your mind that you are on your way to your weight loss goal, and there is a plan in place to get you there. You are not cutting your carbohydrate intake in half simply so you can still eat what you consider good, but so you can prepare your body for the next phase.

If you decide to deviate from this plan, you can rest assured that it is not the end of the world. But it *is* affecting your end results and setting you back. At this point, you are still consuming way more carbohydrates than you need, and your body most likely is storing the excess. However, you are sending a strong message to your mind saying, "I'm in control, and as you can tell. You are not going to continue to force me to eat everything in sight." Once you take control of this situation, you will be ready for week 2, which is an all-out mental war.

All the effort is worth it, and your body is ready to do whatever it is directed to do. Whether it's told to lose weight or gain weight, it will.

Beginning this first step will be fun and challenging. Use it as a *no turning back* tool. Tell yourself, "Now that I've started, there's no turning back. I'm all in!"

Week 2 (7 Days)

This week consists of having no carbohydrates for dinner, while continuing half of your normal carbohydrate intake for breakfast and lunch. Cutting out carbohydrates for an entire meal, in this case dinner, will be a huge step forward in your progress to lose weight. A lot of foods contain carbohydrates, including fruits and vegetables, so for the purpose of this week's challenge, focus on the Enemy List. It consists of the heaviest carbohydrate-filled foods typically served in jails and prisons. Be sure to reference the recipe section of this book to find some new or forgotten ideas on ways to still have an enjoyable meal without carbohydrates.

As mentioned at the start of this section, carbohydrates have benefits, one of which is giving you that full feeling. When you eliminate the foods from the Enemy List for your dinner, your body is going to be very surprised, and your mind is going to tell you things that are not even remotely true. My mind literally tells me that I'm going to starve to death if I don't eat bread. Your stomach will grumble and moan; your every thought will be about some type of carbohydrate-heavy food from the Enemy List.

During this time, it is important to do a few things that will help you tremendously. When your mind is giving you worst-case scenarios if you don't eat the Enemy List foods, remind yourself that the odds of those scenarios are little to none. Instead, give yourself some best-case scenarios. Think of all of the positives that can come from avoiding those noodles. When your stomach is moaning and groaning, it is because your stomach has been used to processing a certain amount of certain types of foods at certain times of the day. Your stomach releases acids and enzymes that break down food. Once the stomach knows your schedule, those acids and enzymes get released right on time, whether you eat or not. Those sounds from your belly are simply the acids and enzymes being released into your digestive tract, looking for food. Those sounds do not mean you're hungry. The other foods you ate for dinner will definitely hold you over until your next meal at breakfast.

Remember, you are currently weaning yourself off of carbohydrates, and your mind and body crave them, but *you* have to be stronger than your cravings. This is how you build self-control. This will positively affect other areas of your life as well.

Week 3 (7 Days)

This week consists of having no carbohydrates for lunch and dinner, while continuing half of your normal carbohydrate intake for breakfast. By now, you most likely have *not* lost any weight. If you have a good job, but for the rest of us, this carbohydrate wean is designed to prepare and train our bodies not to rely on carbohydrates. We will dive into the fat burning directly after week 4 of the Carbohydrate Wean System is over, but for now, it is vital that you follow the Carbohydrate Wean System as described if you want this to work.

By the way, congratulations on making it through week 2 of the plan! The elimination of carbohydrates from dinner is the hardest part of starting the entire program, and where most people struggle or give up. You are doing big things, whether you see it or not. Keep up the good work! This week is a very big one also for two reasons. First, you are eliminating carbohydrate-heavy foods from another entire meal which will compound your missing dinner carbohydrates. Your body will once again start making noises, and your mind will once again bully you. Just do what you practiced last week with positive talk and remind yourself of what those stomach sounds and feelings really are. It will be much easier this time. Second, this week is important to promote habit-building. On average, it takes the human mind 21 days of doing something for it to become a habit. After this week, you will be on day 21 of the Carbohydrate Wean System, teaching your mind and body who is in control and proving that you *can* survive without ridiculous or even moderate amounts of carbohydrate-heavy foods. After this week, you will find that you can do every single thing in this book because the largest hurdles have been cleared.

Eat meats, cheese, vegetables, and fruits for lunch. It is a very light lunch and won't feel like much. That is exactly what we want. Feeling full is what put all of those pounds on us in the first place. Now, all that is necessary is a small portion of zero to no carbohydrate-laden foods.

By the end of this week, your body will begin to look for a new fuel source, and it will find one within you –fat! This means that the fat your body has been storing for future use will now be used, and you will begin to get rid of it. We will discuss this more, but for now, get ready for week 4!

Week 4 (7 Days)

This week consists of having no carbohydrates for breakfast, lunch, or dinner. You made it to week 4, and you should be very proud of yourself, but there is still work to be done. Remember, you will still be consuming carbohydrates through fruits, vegetables, and most foods you eat; our problems come from the foods on the Enemy List. Once again, a small amount of carbohydrates is good for you, just avoid excessive amounts that the body stores as fat.

During this week, you will likely notice a significant difference in your energy levels and your overall well-being. It may feel weird, as if you are not yourself, but once I explain what you are experiencing, you will enjoy the feeling. A lot of people can react negatively to the feelings they experience during this phase; they may get angry or *hangry* (hungry and angry), among other feelings. What you will need to keep in the forefront of your mind is that your body is currently switching fuel sources. For years, sometimes decades, we have been using carbohydrates as our main fuel source. Let's call carbohydrates *unleaded fuel*. Now, after all this time, we are switching to fat as our main fuel source. Let's call it a fat *premium grade*. If you were to suddenly put premium gasoline in a vehicle that has only run on unleaded, there would be a transition as the vehicle gets used to the new fuel, but it would run better when all is said and done. (I know that car people have a lot to say about this analogy; just focus on the fact that we are upgrading to a better fuel, and it will be well worth it.)Trust me, this change takes a lot of getting used to; the way fat burns and the energy you receive from it is very different from carbohydrate energy. It feels purer and more vibrant compared to the carbohydrate energy, which feels duller and more sluggish. When your fat stores are burning up, it really feels as if you are alive, and it's a natural high.

During this week-4 process, you have guided your mind and body onto the path that you want it to go down. Now your entire being is focused on one goal –burn fat! There are still challenges to come, but by getting to this point, you have proven to yourself that you can truly do this. Nothing is out of your reach, and you are now naturally burning up your stored fat. Soon we are going to supercharge that burn, but for now, enjoy your accomplishment!

Drayvon's Carbohydrate Wean Experience

Let's just say I wasn't eating very much while I was out in the free world before my incarceration. And what I did eat was not very healthy.

Once I got to my institution, I ate everything I could. Bread seemed to help me get full and keep me satisfied, so bread became my food of choice. I remember one night I ate 16 slices at dinner! I'm pretty sure that's nearly a whole loaf! My stomach was growing by the week, and my body was storing fat all over. People started calling me *Pan*, which means bread in Spanish. After 8 months, I had gained 32 pounds. It was not a healthy gain either. The joints in my body were screaming at me to do something. I tried to fight through it, but the pain became too much.

I was introduced to the Carbohydrate (Carb) Wean Program by the author of this book, and it truly changed my entire life. It really works! The biggest surprise to me was how everyone said the first week would be so hard, but it really wasn't. I was still able to eat bread and desserts. As the week flew by, it wasn't even an issue. Each week was easier than the previous week. By week 4, I didn't even want carbs; my energy level was so high. I knew that carbohydrates, especially bread, would take all that away. There was no way I was going to allow that to happen!

My weight started to get back to my normal 170 pounds, but I looked different. My stored fat fed my muscles, and I looked really healthy and felt awesome. My joints were no longer yelling at me, and my stomach flattened back out. It was not quite the six-pack I was hoping for, but good enough.

It took about 9 weeks to lose 28 pounds and get back to feeling healthy. The 4-week Carb Wean System jump-started the whole process, and I am so grateful. No matter how much weight you are trying to lose, this system is the best way to get started and make the first big strides to getting to where you want.

Carb Wean Tip

If you have any health issues, be sure to speak with your medical provider before starting any nutrient subtractions or additions. This system, as laid out, is safe on its own with no extreme measures; but a person who is diabetic, for instance, would need carbohydrates during week 4, so an absolute elimination wouldn't work. Be safe and consult with a professional; you can bend and tweak the system to cater to you.

Also, before you begin the carbohydrate wean, really focus on how much you are eating and how you feel an hour afterwards. Do you feel energetic, tired, lazy, sick, happy, angry, etc.? Also, keep track of what you ate and how that certain food made you feel an hour afterwards. Using myself as an example, I notice when I eat spaghetti, I feel fine right afterwards, but an hour later, I don't want to move. If I eat cake with that, I feel an energy spike/sugar high right away, but an hour later, I feel nauseous. This is going to give you a baseline to understand how your body reacts to certain foods and what you can definitely do without.

Your body is a fine-tuned machine, and it's going to make the best out of what you give it. The best thing we can do is give it healthy foods and beverages to allow for optimal performance and health. For example, replace a food that makes you feel not so great with a food that makes you feel good. On spaghetti night, instead of getting the noodles with the meat sauce on top, try the steamed vegetables with the meat sauce on top. Now, that's an impressive improvement! There are more helpful recipes like that in this book.

On the following page is an example of a food journal you can use to get an idea of how food is affecting you. Consider making your own journal to really find out everything you need to know about the impact food has on your life.

Weight Loss Unlocked

Date	Meal	What I Ate	Immediate Mental Feeling	1 Hour Later Physical Feeling	Conclusion
1-1	Cheeseburger pizza, salad, cookies	Cheeseburger pizza, cookies – no salad	Happy, good meal	Bloated, gassy	Try again with salad and no cookies
1-2	Chef salad w/ turkey and egg	Chef salad w/ turkey - no egg	Mediocre, not very filling	Great!	Not eating to get full. I feel good.

CHAPTER TWO

Intermittent Fasting

I know you are ready to supercharge your weight loss goals and speed up your metabolism at the same time. Intermittent fasting is the way to do it. People from all age groups have found many benefits in intermittent fasting, and science is finding new benefits of this all the time.

Intermittent fasting is not a diet or a miserable punishment you must endure. It is actually fun and can easily become a lifestyle. One thing that stands out is the fact that most people who try intermittent fasting find it very difficult to go back to their original eating habits. That alone can help motivate you to find an intermittent fasting system that works for you. What we will do in this section is focus on three intermittent fasting styles and the pros and cons of each one. You'll also learn which style will give you a head start plus a positive life lesson. I want you to read this section of the book at least twice before you begin so you really understand what you are going to be looking at and how you will navigate the terrain. There are so many benefits to intermittent fasting; I want you to experience them all! I have been intermittent fasting steadily for about one year, and it is truly one of the best things I have ever done in my life.

Breakfast, the *worst* meal of the day for those of us trying to lose weight, has been eliminated from my diet as I now only eat two complete meals per day. The first meal I eat is lunch, typically between 12 p.m. and 1 p.m. The second and final meal is dinner, which can be any time before 8 p.m. After 8 p.m., I do not eat again until lunchtime the next day. This means I have an eight-hour window to eat each day. In total, I am also fasting for sixteen hours each day, which, as we will dive into, you will see how this version of fasting can scorch your fat stores.

The biggest surprise I've experienced since beginning intermittent fasting is that I've increased muscle mass and lowered my body fat at the same time. One example is that my jiggly arms are now pretty solid. I am not saying they look like The Rock's arms, but the fat that was there is gone and staying gone.

Sometimes on this weight loss journey, we look at the scale to give us all the answers we need, but it simply can't. Just as in the example I mentioned about my arms becoming solid, that transition could still have me at the same weight, even though I have made huge progress.

Another surprise I had was that my explosiveness during workouts increased substantially. My bench-press weight went up 60 pounds, and my leg press weight went up 50 pounds within sixty days. My stamina also increased, and I noticed that I was finishing my one-hour workouts in about forty minutes. I work out five days a week, so that twenty minutes each day adds up to around 100 minutes a week! If you add it all up, I'm much leaner, much stronger, and more explosive than I ever imagined. I also eat less and have more time to work with.

You might be asking now, "Is this for real –skip breakfast? That's not good, is it? Are there really benefits to fasting for 16 hours? Why would a person do that? Is there danger involved with this? What does science say about this?" Well, lucky for you, we will discuss each of these questions so you can decide if this is right for you. All of your questions are good questions and valid, and I felt the same skepticism at first. But after my own personal research, which I will share with you, I am a true believer and have never felt better. I have done some pretty crazy stuff when it comes to losing weight, but this is not one of them. Intermittent fasting is the real deal. You can easily implement this style of fasting into your life, and the benefits to your health are numerous.

In this section, we will go over the three most common styles of intermittent fasting. We will break it down from the easiest to the hardest and the pros and cons for each. As you read through each one, think about your typical day and when you are feeling the hungriest. For me, it is the late afternoon and early evening. This will help you choose the right intermittent fasting style for you and give you a chance to pick your own time frames. You will truly enjoy intermittent fasting, and you will love the benefits.

What's Intermittent Fasting?

Intermittent fasting is not in any way a diet. Intermittent fasting is a pattern of consuming food on a schedule. The way you plan your meals determines how much fat you burn. Changing *when* you eat instead of *what* you eat is the foundation of intermittent fasting. Obviously, you'll need to stay away from foods on the Enemy List to maximize results, but with intermittent fasting, you do get a little bit of wiggle room without falling off the cliff.

The most common question I get asked is, "What difference would it make to change *when* I eat?" Well, the first reason is that it is a great way to burn fat and get lean without having to go on a stressful diet where you can barely eat, you get frustrated, and give up. The second reason is that you can keep your caloric intake (calories) nearly the same as it was before you ever started intermittent fasting! You can actually go a little bigger with your meals because you have a short time frame to consume your meals. All in all, changing when you eat will give your body the opportunity to burn stored fat while still allowing you to keep your muscle mass.

Clearly, the number one reason that a person starts intermittent fasting is to lose weight. We will go over how exactly intermittent fasting leads to weight loss in the upcoming pages, but I do want to point this out. Prison puts a lot of dampers on a lot of plans, but intermittent fasting is by far one of the easiest strategies you can use to your advantage for taking off unwanted fat and keeping good muscle. Intermittent fasting puts you in the driver's seat and lets you be in full control of everything, and it requires just a tiny behavior change. As a matter of fact, it just requires fighting a temptation over one meal a day. This is the best news of all because it means it's so easy, we can do it in prison, and it is one aspect of your life you can have power over again. The difference it will make in your life will be felt soon after starting and every day after that. Each day it gets easier until it is normal, and you don't even think about it. Only you can begin this, and I hope you start soon because your body wants to burn that fat up. That's why your body stores it. Let's get into that.

Intermittent Fasting: How in the World Does it Work?

This may be my favorite part of the book. This is where we get into how intermittent fasting burns fat as fuel! To really learn how intermittent fasting relates to fat burning and weight loss, we need to first learn the distinction between the *fed phase* and the *fasted phase*. These two phases are the keys to unlocking your fat-burning potential. Your body immediately enters the fed phase/fed state when it is absorbing or digesting any food you have fed to your body. Usually, the fed phase begins when you start eating and will continue for three to six hours while your body processes and digests the food you just consumed. Depending on your metabolism, the fed phase can even last up to eight hours.

While you are in the fed phase, it is nearly impossible for your body to burn fat because your insulin levels are extremely high, and your body is dedicated to digesting the food as efficiently as possible. When the fed phase period is finished, your body immediately enters the **post-absorptive** phase. This is a very technical way of saying that your body is done processing food. The post-absorptive phase lasts for an average of ten hours after your last meal. When this ten-hour post-absorptive phase is over, that is when your body goes into the fasted phase. Now your body can start burning fat. Your body has a lot of really useful ways to burn fat, and now that your insulin levels are low with no food to digest, your body will burn your stored fat until you eat again. The reason you have this fat is because your body stores it for energy use in the future, as fat is fuel. When your body is in the fasted phase, it can burn fat that was inaccessible while your body was in the fed phase.

Seeing as how we don't come into the fasted phase for 10 hours after the last meal we ate, it is uncommon for many of us (most of us) to enter this intense fat scorching state. I mean, before I began intermittent fasting, I couldn't ever remember going 10 hours without eating. But once you start doing this, you'll never stop. Many times, the battle is mental, and you will be asleep for most of your post-absorptive phase, sometimes even into your fasted phase. Those ten hours will be nothing compared to the lifetime of benefits you'll earn. Getting into the fasted phase and allowing your body to access and burn stored fat is easier than you ever imagined.

You, like most people who begin intermittent fasting, will lose fat without changing how much you eat, what you eat, or even your exercise schedule. Being in the fasted phase for even just a few hours a day puts your body in a fat-incinerating mode that you would seldom ever make it to during a typical eating program.

So, what are the benefits? Fat burning is awesome, but there are a few other reasons to start intermittent fasting. Here are two:

- Your day is simpler.
- You can live a longer life using intermittent fasting!

I am a big believer in forming positive habits, reducing stress, and using life hacks. Intermittent fasting checks all of these boxes and simplifies your life. You will enjoy the way your day flows as you wake up and don't have to worry about what to eat for breakfast. When I wake up in the morning, I chug a sixteen-ounce tumbler of water and don't even think about food. My entire morning is free, and my body is either entering or already in the fasted phase, and I can literally feel the fat being burned and used as energy.

I truly enjoy cooking and eating. Preparing food, no matter what it is, is meditative for me. Whipping up a few meals a day never really bothered me, because I had a chance to meditate and eat some of my world-class cooking. The benefit of intermittent fasting is that it allows me to subtract one meal, which means I don't have to plan this meal, prepare this meal, and eat this meal. That is such a stress reliever and makes my life a lot simpler. I really appreciate that.

In the scientific community, they have long known that restricting calories is a way to lengthen a person's life. Taking a logical look at that point, it makes a lot of sense. If you are giving your body the impression that you're starving, your body will find a way to lengthen your life. I can already hear you, "Who wants to starve themselves just to live longer?"

You won't be starving; your body just thinks it is. Also, speaking for myself, I want to live for as long as I can, and missing a meal a day doesn't seem like too harsh of a price to pay for that reward. The best news of the day is that intermittent fasting initiates so many of the same mechanisms for lengthening a person's life as restricting calories. What this means for you is that you receive the benefits of an expanded life without the drama of starving!

In the 1940's, scientists learned that intermittent fasting lengthened the life in lab mice. In the early 2000's, scientists discovered that alternate-day intermittent fasting directly led to extended life spans. Once you start intermittent fasting and start feeling and seeing the benefits of it, you'll want to continue your success and live a longer life, it will be all worth it.

You may actually lower your risk of cancer. Although it is debated within the scientific community, the data out currently looks very promising. There definitely needs to be more research and studies in this arena along with experimentation to find what exact relationship exists between fasting and cancer.

A recently released study of less than fifty cancer patients made the suggestion that the side effects of chemotherapy might be lessened by certain types of fasting before receiving treatment. This revelation is dually held up by a separate study that incorporated alternate day fasting with certain cancer patients, which came to the conclusion that fasting prior to chemotherapy treatment resulted in a higher cure rate and a lower amount of lives lost. All in all, this in-depth analysis of several studies on the relationship between diseases and fasting has shown that fasting appears to reduce the risk of cancer and that is an extremely good reason to begin a lifestyle of intermittent fasting.

Intermittent fasting is effortless compared to dieting. There are many reasons diets fail, but the most common reason isn't because we switch to the improper foods, it is because most of us don't actually stick to the dieting plan for a long period of time. This makes it not an issue of nutrition, but rather an issue of behavioral habits. This is the good news! This means your main goal is to change your habits and intermittent fasting is the best way to do that. Once you make these changes, intermittent fasting really breaks free and stands out as the beacon of hope it is. You begin to see how utterly easy it is to implement once you get past the notion that you have to eat all of the time. One example is a study that found intermittent fasting was a very effective strategy for consistent weight loss in adults who are obese. In its conclusion, the study states that "individuals quickly adapt" to a routine of intermittent fasting. This means that your body is already tuned for a program like this. Your mind is the only naysayer, but after a short time, your mind will see the ease of intermittent fasting and get in line.

Dr. Michael Eades, PhD, said some very important things after trying intermittent fasting. I'd like to quote him on his interpretation of intermittent fasting versus a diet. "Diets are easy in contemplation, difficult in execution. Intermittent fasting is just the opposite. It is difficult in the contemplation but easy in the execution."

Most of us have thought about going on a diet. When we find a diet that appeals to us, it seems as if it will be a breeze to do. But when we get into the nitty-gritty of it, it becomes tough. For example, I stay on a low-carb diet almost all the time. But if I think about going on a low-fat diet, it looks easy. I think about bagels, whole wheat bread, jelly, mashed potatoes, corn, bananas by the dozen, etc., all of which sound appealing. But if I were to embark on such a low-fat diet, I would soon tire of it and wish I could have meat and eggs. So, a diet is easy to consider but not so easy in the long-term application.

Intermittent fasting is hard in contemplation, there is no doubt. "You go without food for 24 hours?" people would ask incredulously when I explained what I was doing, "I could never do that." But once you start, it's a snap. No worries about what and where to eat for one or two out of three meals per day. It's a great liberator; your food expenditures plummet, and you're not particularly hungry. According to Dr. Eades, "Although it's tough to overcome the idea of going without food, once you begin the regimen, nothing could be easier."

In my humble opinion, the ease and simplistic nature of intermittent fasting is the top reason to give it a shot. It provides a wide array of health benefits without changing too much of your lifestyle. Rather than having to plan meals, buy certain foods, and deprive yourself of anything good, you are simply going to eliminate one meal, either breakfast or dinner, from your day. How beautiful is that?

Intermittent Fasting Styles

Now we will get into some examples of different intermittent fasting schedules to find out which one is best for you. If you are considering giving intermittent fasting a try, these will be your best bet for beginning an intermittent fasting lifestyle.

Weekly Intermittent Fasting

One of the smoothest transitions from your regular eating into intermittent fasting is weekly intermittent fasting. It is the best way to get started because you only do it once per week or once per month. This style of fasting has already been shown to lead to many of the benefits we have discussed regarding your health. This means that even if you don't use it to reduce your calorie intake, there are still many health benefits. The following illustration shows one example of how a weekly intermittent fasting schedule might look.

Chart of Intermittent Fasting

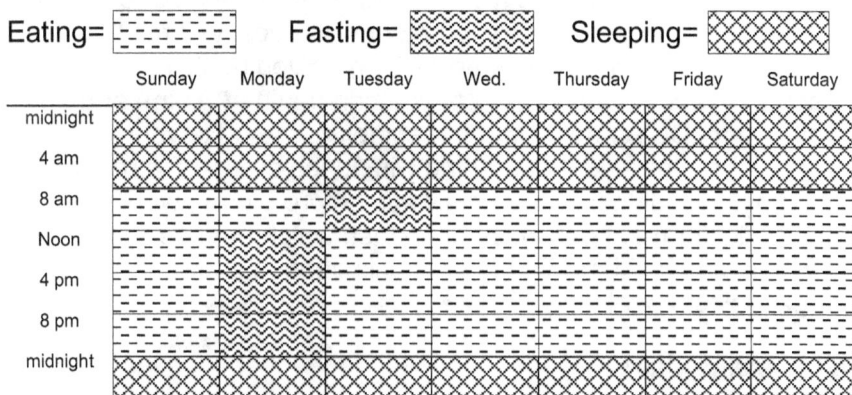

Using this chart, lunch on Monday is your final meal for the day. You then fast until lunchtime on Tuesday. This schedule definitely has the advantage of letting you eat meals every day of the week while still receiving the health benefits of fasting for a 24-hour period. It's also a sure thing that you won't lose very much weight with this style of intermittent fasting because you are only cutting out 1 or 2 meals per week. The purpose of weekly intermittent fasting is to prove to yourself that you can survive for 24 hours without food. This style will also help cleanse your system and improve your metabolism. It's a crash course in intermittent fasting and your own personal starter kit.

In the past, as recently as 3 weeks ago, I've done a 24-hour fast. There are multiple variations and choices for fitting a 24-hour fast into your schedule. For instance, after a big meal, a spread, or a holiday meal are some of the best times to do an unscheduled 24-hour fast to go along with your weekly intermittent fast.

Daily Intermittent Fasting

This is by far my favorite intermittent fasting style, if I can even call it that anymore, since it's just part of my day, part of my life now. I follow the Leangains model of intermittent fasting most of the time, which incorporates an 8-hour eating zone followed by a 16-hour fast. This can also be called an eight-sixteen. This style of intermittent fasting was made popular by Martin Berkhan, who is part of Leangains.com and the place the name originated from.

Whenever you want to start your eight-hour eating zone is definitely up to you, just try to be consistent daily. It really doesn't matter when you start as long as you do it. You can start at 9 a.m. and end at 5 p.m., or you can begin at 3 p.m. and end at 11 p.m. Do whatever works best for you and fits your schedule. I learned that starting with lunch around 1 p.m. and ending after dinner, which is always before 9 p.m., works perfectly for me. I only miss breakfast, which I am perfectly okay with. It's no big deal. The following illustration shows the Leangains model.

Leangains Chart

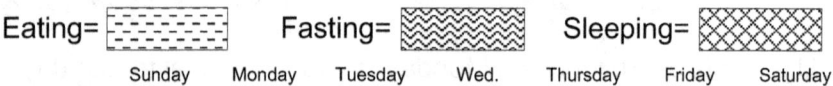

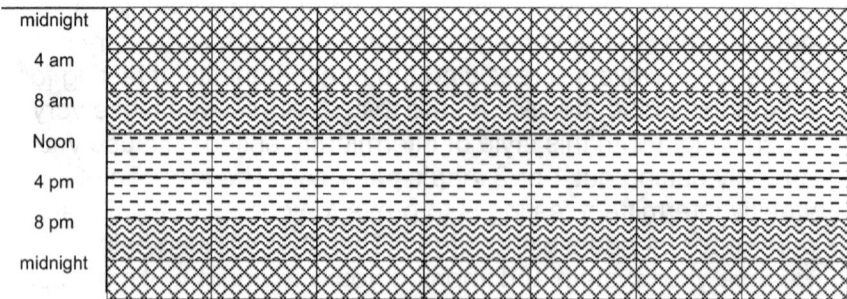

Eating=   Fasting=   Sleeping=

	Sunday	Monday	Tuesday	Wed.	Thursday	Friday	Saturday
midnight							
4 am							
8 am							
Noon							
4 pm							
8 pm							
midnight							

Since daily intermittent fasting is done each and every day, it creates a healthy habit and is very easy to maintain on the schedule of your choosing. At this moment in time, you are most likely eating your meals and snacks around the same time every day. You may not have noticed, but if you think about it you go to chow at roughly the same time and finish before a certain time, seven days a week. You also reach into your storage box between certain TV shows or after specific line movements, you just haven't thought much about it. I used to think, "I'm eating because I'm hungry *now*." But once I started logging my snacks, I saw a pattern: after work, 8 p.m. and 11 p.m. These were my snack times. With daily intermittent fasting, it's the exact opposite. You simply learn not to eat at specific times. It is surprisingly easy!

One of the possible setbacks of daily intermittent fasting is the fact that, because you usually remove at least one if not two meals from your day, it starts to become very difficult to attempt to get the same number of calories your body is used to during the day. Said differently, it can be tough to train yourself to eat larger meals on a consistent basis, fewer times a day. This results in a lot of people who practice daily intermittent fasting finding themselves *losing weight*! I don't know what else could be better!

The final thing I'll say about daily intermittent fasting is that while I've been practicing this style of fasting for about a year, I'm not religious about my diet. Daily intermittent fasting helped me build healthy habits that direct my behavior 95% of the time. This means for the other 5% of the time, I can do whatever I want. When the pizza and cookies call my name and it's outside of my fasting schedule, I can eat it knowing that it won't throw me off course because I've maintained my schedule for the last month. Don't torture yourself; treat yourself here and there. It will be funny, though, because a lot of junk food becomes unattractive once you go without it for a while. Just don't go back to eating it every day. You'll love daily intermittent fasting.

Alternate Day Intermittent Fasting

Alternate-day intermittent fasting is one of the harder versions of intermittent fasting. This style of fasting involves fasting for much longer periods on alternate days throughout the week. If you look at the sample chart that follows, you will eat dinner on Monday evening, and then you will not eat any food until Tuesday night. Make sure to get at least 24 hours, if not more, before eating your meal on Tuesday night. Once you eat on Tuesday you can continue to eat all day on Wednesday, however, you will start a new 24-hour fasting cycle again on Wednesday night.

Alternate day intermittent fasting allows you to get at least 24 hours of fasting on a consistent basis while allowing you to eat at least one meal every day. This type of fasting seems to be the most popular form of fasting for those who don't have an exercise regimen because the 24-hour fasts can make up for the lack of exercise. A huge benefit of alternate-day fasting is that you get a much longer time in the fasted phase than you would with the daily intermittent fasting style. This means you will receive greater benefits than if you use another style of fasting.

Now that I have discussed some of the pros involved in alternate-day intermittent fasting, let's examine a con to this method. When using this type of fasting, you will not be getting many nutrients. Even on the days you do eat, it will be hard to compensate for that loss on your alternate day. Based on my experimentation, training yourself to consistently eat more is the most difficult part of alternate-day fasting. A person might be able to stuff himself for a single meal, but teaching oneself to do that every single day of the week takes a little bit of strategic planning, a little cooking, and consistent eating. The outcome of this is that many people who try alternate day fasting end up losing weight, but also deprive themselves of nutrients unless they develop a plan to make up for those nutrients within their eating time frames. Fruits and vegetables are a great way to load your body with nutrients. It will be very difficult to eat enough food to stay properly nourished, so make sure you have a plan before starting alternate-day fasting.

Alternate Day Fasting Chart

Eating= [pattern]   Fasting= [pattern]   Sleeping= [pattern]

	Sunday	Monday	Tuesday	Wed.	Thursday	Friday	Saturday
midnight	Sleeping	Sleeping	Sleeping	Sleeping	Sleeping	Sleeping	Sleeping
4 am	Sleeping	Sleeping	Sleeping	Sleeping	Sleeping	Sleeping	Sleeping
8 am	(blank)	Eating	Fasting	Eating	Fasting	Eating	Fasting
Noon	(blank)	Eating	Fasting	Eating	Fasting	Eating	Fasting
4 pm	(blank)	Eating	Fasting	Eating	Fasting	Eating	Fasting
8 pm	(blank)	Fasting	Eating	Fasting	Eating	Fasting	Eating
midnight	(blank)	Sleeping	Sleeping	Sleeping	Sleeping	Sleeping	Sleeping

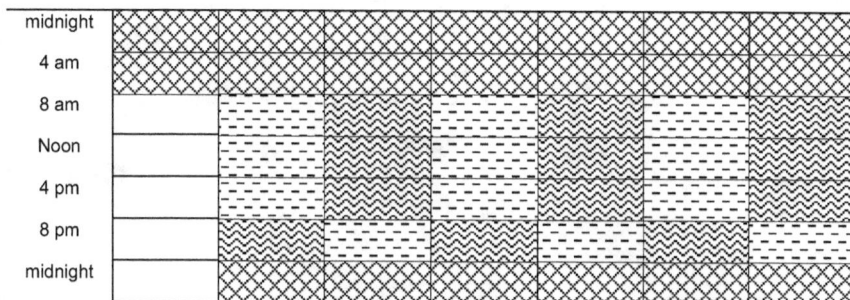

*Sunday is left blank to allow opposite switch each week.

"Storms make trees grow deeper roots."
– Claude McDonald

Some days, we all feel like everything is falling apart, and it will never get better. But how many times have we thought that? So many times, it happens, and we always come out on top. You might think you are too old or too big or too _____ (you fill in the blank) to start losing weight. Treat it like every other trial and tribulation in your life and push through it. You will be stronger than ever before and so proud of yourself!

CHAPTER THREE

Common Questions & Concerns

During my weight-loss journey, intermittent fasting was the most impactful behavioral change I made. As I worked with other inmates and staff on their health goals, they had their own concerns and questions about intermittent fasting. I thought I'd share some with you because you might be thinking the same question or having the same concerns.

- Q. I'm a woman. Does intermittent fasting affect me differently?

- A. Well, I'm not a woman, so all I can tell you is what I've seen in other women who have fasted intermittently and the research I've done. I have read that women may be able to find a wider window of opportunity for eating, which would be much more favorable while doing an intermittent fasting schedule. Whereas men will usually fast for 16 hours and eat for 8 hours each day on the daily intermittent fasting, women can find much better results by fasting for 14 hours and eating for 10 hours. That's an extra 2 hours! The thing I advise most to everyone, not only women, is to try what works for you. Your body will let you know.

- Q. How on earth do you skip breakfast?

- A. I never miss breakfast. Breakfast is my favorite meal of the day. I simply eat my breakfast at 1:00 in the afternoon, every day. Plus, if you eat a large dinner the night before, you will be very surprised by how much energy you have when you wake up in the morning. Most of the concerns that come with people contemplating intermittent fasting are drawn from the constant barrage of information that is pounded into our heads by the multi-billion-dollar breakfast companies telling us that we need to eat breakfast. They insist that it is the most important meal of the day. Now that I understand the three phases of consumption: fed, post-absorptive, and fasted, I realize that I'm literally waking up in a fat-burning state or just a few hours or less from entering one. It dawned on me that breakfast is the most *harmful* meal of the day. If you don't give yourself at least 16 hours from your evening meal to your next day's meal, eating anything will immediately pull you out of the post-absorptive and/or the fasted phase and reset you back to the fed phase, where you burn no fat storage. The science doesn't back up the breakfast companies, and neither does my personal experience.

- Q. I read in a magazine that I should eat every three hours. What about that?

- A. Yes, there are many magazine articles that say that you should eat six small meals a day, every three hours, or something close to three hours. If you are wondering why this was a popular idea for a while, here is the reason: when your body is processing food, it's burning calories. This resulted in the idea that the multiple meals strategy would ensure that you would burn more calories during the day if you ate more frequently. The outcome would ultimately be that you would lose weight. Here is the problem with that: the total amount of calories a person burns is directly related to the size of the meal your body is trying to process. This means, for example, as your body digests six smaller meals that amount to 2,200 calories, your body will use the same amount of energy as if you ate two meals that are larger and total 1,100 calories each. Either way, you burn the same number of calories. It wouldn't matter if you received your calories from fifteen meals or one meal; if the calorie count is the same, you get the same result.

- Q. Won't I die if I don't eat for 24 hours?

- A. Truthfully, I'm a firm believer that the mental aspect of fasting is the biggest barrier that stops people from getting started or completing a successful intermittent fasting schedule. Intermittent fasting is not very hard, but your mind will tell you otherwise. I'll give you a few reasons as to why intermittent fasting isn't as abstract as you might be thinking. Intermittent fasting has been around for a very long time, and it really works! Many religions and groups have practiced intermittent fasting for hundreds of years. Health and medical professionals have also discerned the many health benefits that humans have received from intermittent fasting over our entire known history. This lets us know that intermittent fasting isn't some new, hot trend. It's been around as long as we have. Wow, that's amazing!

Another reason that intermittent fasting seems so foreign to most people is simply due to the fact that there is a huge effort by big companies to silence the intermittent fasting lifestyle. Nobody is going to make money by telling you not to eat their company's food product. Put differently, intermittent fasting isn't a good marketing strategy or profitable; therefore, you are not exposed to the issue enough for it to be something that doesn't sound extreme, even though it is normal.

The third reason I'll mention is that you have most likely fasted several times, but you didn't know it! Remember that time you slept in late on Saturday morning and then had brunch? Most people do this every weekend! Think about it. We usually eat our last meal of the day on Friday night and then don't eat again on Saturday until around lunchtime, sometimes later. There's your 12-16-hour fast, and it didn't even cross your mind.

Lastly, my advice to all is to do one 24-hour period of fasting, even if intermittent fasting is not something you plan on doing. The reason is that you will prove to yourself that you won't die if you don't eat for a day. As you battle with your mind, you will shut down that voice in your head and show yourself that this is something you *can* do!

- Q. Where else can I learn about intermittent fasting?

- A. A good place to start is by rereading this section. Once you finish, you can have a family member or friend send you some information from the internet. The best way to learn is by experimenting to see what actually works for you.

Kristen Mancinelli has a book titled *Jump Start Ketosis*. She writes about how intermittent fasting will put your body into a state of ketosis, where it burns fat instead of glucose for energy. It's a very detailed guide.

I really hope you start intermittent fasting and stick with it until it becomes your new normal. You will feel so much better and healthier; your days will be less stressful and simplified. That's it in a nutshell. Just make sure to talk to your medical provider first.

Intermittent Whaaa?

I will never forget the day my buddy told me that he wanted me to try intermittent fasting with him. First of all, I don't like big words. Secondly, I love to eat, way too much. He was so intent on doing it that I told him okay, but just for a week. All we had to do was skip breakfast for seven days. I was not happy about that, but I figured the menu would repeat itself, and missing breakfast for a week might do me some good.

I won't lie, the first morning was not fun. It was pancake day, and I almost said, "forget this", in so many words. Until lunchtime, I thought I would starve to death, but surely, I wouldn't. I was so happy eating lunch, and dinner was even better.

On day 2, breakfast was much easier because I now knew it was only a matter of hours before I could eat again. I felt really good and went for a light jog. I noticed that I felt a lot lighter without all of that breakfast in my belly. I also felt like I had a ton of energy. This was one of the best mornings I've ever had. Not only was my body feeling great, but my mental clarity was really good.

By day 3, and every day after that, there has been nothing to worry about because I feel better and my attitude is positive. I have lost 32 pounds, and I can lift more weight than I could when I was bigger. As I write this, I am on day 345; 20 more days will be a whole year!

Intermittent fasting sounded crazy at first, let's be real, but it was worth it. I also outlasted my friend who wanted to be fasting partners! Oh well, when you really want something, you have to go for it. You can too!

– Lindin P.

CHAPTER FOUR

Water Works!
What You Need To Know
About H20

Water is life. Without it, nothing could grow. Nothing could sustain life. Everything would die. So, the question is, why are you barely drinking any water at all? Well, we are going to change that together, and you will be so happy that you did! Tell your cellmate, tell your boss at work that it's going to get a little wild with you and the restroom, but just for a week or two, as your body adjusts to the massive water increase you are about to undergo for the next 30 days. This is another healthy habit you will love yourself for starting.

Water and Your Health

First, let's look at water and how it affects our health. Most people in the criminal justice system in this country suffer from aches and pains, fatigue, skin disorders, and constipation. It might be hard to believe, but most of the time, all of these ailments are brought about simply by a lack of water. We as inmates guzzle coffee by the gallon along with soda pop, juice, and sweet tea. Regular old water for most of us is just too boring or, worse, nasty.

It is time to get past that and realize that you really *need* water. Most of the inmates and staff that I worked with on weight loss goals informed me right off the bat that they didn't drink water. Right after that, they would assure me that there's nothing to worry about because they were getting enough liquids throughout the day. When I went a little deeper to get a better understanding as to what these "liquids" were, you guessed it – coffee, soda pop, juices, and iced tea with sugar. A lot of people who consume large quantities of supplements, usually vitamins, every day, take them with at least a cup of coffee or a soda pop. Well, it is no wonder they are having issues! Their bodies are not being allowed to operate properly because they're not getting pure water.

Think about it; your body is made up of approximately 75% water. Other than oxygen, water is the most important in terms of our survival. Water regulates body temperature and flushes out wastes and toxins. As for your muscles, joints, and bones, water acts as a shock absorber. Water cleanses the body on the outside and on the inside. Water moves proteins, minerals, sugars, and vitamins around the body for proper assimilation. In order to function at your tiptop, peak performance, you must drink water in the right amounts.

A lot of people I met had issues with bloating, water retention, and edema. After they started drinking a lot of water daily, most of their issues vanished! When trying to lose weight, it is important to remember that water helps suppress hunger cravings. In order to keep your body's complex systems maintained and functioning properly, drinking clean, good water each and every day is the perfect start. I will discuss the proper recommended amount of water each person needs each day, but for now, the average recommended amount is 6 to 8 glasses per day. If possible, drink more than this.

Since you most likely haven't been drinking much water, this sudden increase may seem like a lot to deal with. But you are going to have to start at some point, so dive in. If you are allowed an apple in your cell, try throwing a slice in the glass of water to help with the benefits of cleansing. Additionally, water is a bit easier to drink with a hint of flavor. This seems to work well for a lot of people who used to think that it was impossible to drink more water. Before they know it, they are running around with a pitcher of water everywhere they go. This also goes to show how much better life is simply by drinking more water; now they can't seem to put the water down!

- There are different types of water. Once you get going on increasing your water intake, a common concern naturally becomes, "What is the best water for me to drink?" Well, as inmates, our choices are limited mostly to tap water, but things are changing; we'll go over the top four most commonly consumed types of water so we can learn the benefits of each. Most of our tap water contains chlorine, fluoride, and many other chemicals that are used to treat tap water. These are harmless, but it is important to know. This may help to clarify other types of water.

- Distilled water: This is one of the most famous types of water. Most people believe that distilled water is the only way to go. I'm not here to argue, but I would respectfully disagree. Yes, it is a fact that distilled water is by far the purest water offered to us because it is demineralized (lacks minerals). That is not what we are looking for on our quest for optimum health. The human body craves minerals found in water. Distilled water is an excellent detoxifier and an even better cleanser. However, it's not nutritious as it is demineralized.

- Mineral water: Mineral water typically comes from a natural spring and contains minerals from that spring. The tastes vary depending on the season. The natural minerals in mineral water are directly responsible for aiding digestion and bowel movements.

- Filtered water: When bottled water is not in your plans, you can use a water filter. Some prisons have the filter attached to the common sink. Some pitchers now come equipped with filtration devices that purify the water as the pitcher fills up. These are two really important inventions that are helping even third-world countries where water needs to be filtered, so they can definitely help you. This is something you can work on in your facility to help everyone out.

- Sparkling water: Sparkling water is not typically available in most prisons, but I see the market growing, and I believe it will be a soda alternative soon. Sparkling water comes from natural carbonation in underground springs. Most of the brands we see today are artificially enhanced in carbonation by CO_2 to help boost and maintain that fizz we all love.

Regardless of the type of water you decide on, the main thing to remember is that you must be mindful of the amount of water you consume every day. Just because you feel thirsty, that is not a reliable sign that your body needs water. During the course of activity, you can lose over a quart of water before you even feel a hint of thirst.

One other thing I keep in the front of my mind is that coffee, tea, soda pop –all caffeinated beverages are diuretics. This means that they increase your body's need for pure water. Put differently, these caffeinated beverages dehydrate you, which is the opposite of what we're trying to do here. It is safe to say that if you are serious about improving your overall health, caffeine does not belong. But if you can't go without it, simply make sure you compensate by drinking 2 cups of water for every cup of caffeinated beverage consumed.

Benefits of Water

The past 15 years have really changed the way we deal with water. The substance that makes up most of our body, makes up most of our planet, deserves the opportunity to be boasted about, and that's what we will do now. Here are just a few of the benefits of drinking more water every day.

- You feel better, physically and mentally. When I start feeling irritated and stressed out. I'm going to drink a full cup of water. You can try this too. It is an opportunity for me to get away, reset, and hydrate myself –3 birds, 1 stone! Many studies have linked even slight hydration to improving mood. The irritation you're feeling might have nothing to do with your coworker. It could simply be that you are in need of water. Approximately 80% of your brain tissue is made of water! When you are dehydrated, your mind and body are literally stressed. Water is how you ease this stress.

  When you feel a headache or muscle twitch starting, try drinking a couple of cups of water. Studies show that complete relief is achievable within thirty minutes to an hour after drinking two cups of water. Once water becomes a regular part of your life, your chances of preventing future headaches and twitches/spasms are huge. Always keep a cup or pitcher near you and drink often.

- Water is our best friend when it comes to boosting our energy levels. Feeling tired is one of the first red flags of dehydration. Also, dehydration can impair attention span, memory, and even focus. If you notice yourself drifting off or having trouble concentrating, you've got it, drink more water! That feeling of being depleted and wiped out is usually connected directly to dehydration. Drinking that extra water can help your heart pump blood throughout your body more efficiently. Water consumption is also going to allow oxygen to travel more effectively through your body by way of red blood cells, along with nutrients that are necessary for peak performance.

- Lose weight with water! Yes, I know this is what you've been waiting for, but I do want to talk about the physical and mental benefits first. The first thing you need to do is drink a cup of water before each meal. This not only makes you feel full before you even take your first bite, but it will also make you eat less. Drinking water before the meal is also one of the top 3 ways to speed up your metabolism. Ice water has been shown to accelerate this process. As your body has to work a little harder to heat up the cold water, you automatically burn more calories.

- Cleanse your system! One of the best ways to keep your bowel movements regular and emptying your bladder frequently is with water. Water does this by flushing waste through your digestive tract. Water helps break down waste particles and helps them move along smoothly. When your body is dehydrated, it will absorb all of the water in your digestive tract, leaving your colon completely dry and making it very difficult to have a bowel movement. That is never fun. Water will also bind to fiber to help things get moving.

Kidney health and water go hand in hand. Water eases the burden on the kidneys. The number of people diagnosed with kidney stones continues to rise. One of the most likely reasons for this is that children and adults are not consuming enough water. Water dilutes the minerals and salts in your urinary tract that form the crystals known as kidney stones. These stones cannot form when the urine is diluted. Your chances of kidney stones almost disappear when you drink lots of water!

- Water helps your workouts! Along with the energy-increasing benefits we discussed earlier, water will help you with your exercise program and day-to-day activities. Water does this by getting into your joints to keep them flexible and slick. This lubrication of your joints is a key part in helping you move more fluidly (pun intended) and will keep you from injuring your joints. Water also helps prevent your muscles from cramping by providing them with proper hydration and oxygen.

  It's really not an extreme hurdle to overcome to drink water before, during, and after your workout. The connection between water and exercise is pretty clear. Here's something to think about: regardless of whether you're working out in the July heat or the January cold, we all need water, period. It is the same year-round. In the summer, we are sweating so much that we lose most of our water; therefore, we must replenish the water supply in our bodies. The winter cold is a little different because we plow through our body's water reserve, but it is due to the many layers of clothes which still increase sweating. The sweat is not always as visible in the cold because it is turned to steam and evaporated quickly, just like when you can see your breath. This can be deceptive, and you might think you don't sweat much. But you do so, make sure to stay hydrated in the cold weather, along with the hot summers.

As you can see, water is extremely important to overall health, and there is no substitute. Science continues to discover more and more about the physical and mental benefits of water. This is what our early ancestors drank and kept them alive during times of famine. Our bodies can go nearly two months without food, but a person cannot go more than 3 days without water. Think about that, and you will start to understand the significance of water in your life! With all that said, it's time for your H_2O challenge.

30-Day H₂O Gallon Challenge

Now that you are refreshed with the benefits of water, it's time to start your 30-Day H₂O Gallon Challenge! I'm pretty sure you know that you are going to drink a gallon of water every day for thirty days. I am so excited for you! Just to be clear, you *are* going to drink one gallon of water every day for 30 days.

First things first, let's figure out what you'll be drinking out of so you know what will equal a gallon. The top three water containers that I've seen in prison are:

- The 2-Quart Pitcher
- The 16-Ounce Tumbler
- The 8-Ounce Cup

Now let's figure out the math. Don't worry, we will do it together.

1 Gallon (Liquid) =
4 Quarts =
3.785 Liters =
128 Ounces

In order to consume a gallon of water, use a:

- 2-quart pitcher = drink 2 full pitchers each day
- 16-ounce tumbler = drink 8 filled-to-the-top tumbler cups each day
- 8-ounce cup = drink 16 filled to the top cups each day

This is a lot easier than it looks. What I did was split the total down the middle, so if what you have is an 8-ounce cup, you have to drink 16 cups (sixteen times). If you split the 16 down the middle, now you have 8 and 8, for a total of 16 cups. Focus on drinking the first 8 cups before lunchtime. Now you have the rest of the day until you go to sleep to drink the other 8 cups. If you can, get a pitcher. Drink one full pitcher before lunch and the second pitcher throughout the rest of the day. It's that easy.

Your body will be stunned by this new development and will be sending you to the restroom quite often. This will go on for about a week, but stick to the plan. It will become less and less until you are still consuming a gallon, but you will be using the restroom normally. This 30-Day H₂O Gallon Challenge is going to transform you in so many great ways. Physically, you are going to feel better and flush your body free of harmful bacteria, cleaning your digestive and urinary tracts, and oxygenating your entire body. That's just for starters; mentally, you will be hydrated, so your mood will be gone, and you'll be happier. You will also be proving to yourself that you can do anything you put your mind to!

One thing I noticed is that when I'm chugging water, my mind will tell me to stop drinking so much water, and it would be followed by an immediate physical sensation. One day, I decided to block the thought the minute it happened, and I ignored the physical sensation in my stomach that was saying, "Stop!" The mind plays so many tricks on us and will even induce pain or pleasure to prove to you that the thought is real. If you have ever jogged, your mind will start telling you that you are tired, you are hurting, you'll die if you keep jogging, etc. But every jogger will tell you that if you just ignore these thoughts and the accompanying pain, it completely goes away because it was never real. Your body is in control of processing the water, not your mind, so ignore the thoughts to stop drinking and keep chugging along!

Use the following chart to keep track of your water progress each day. Each box is a day of your challenge. Every day you finish a pitcher, a tumbler, or a cup, make a tally mark. Pitcher drinkers need 2 tallies per day, tumbler drinkers need 8 tallies per day, and 8-ounce cup drinkers need 16 tallies per day. All you have to do is do it, and it will happen! It's go time!

Water Challenge Calendar

Water Challenge Calendar

Make a tally for each container finished: 2-quart pitcher = 2 per day;
16-ounce tumbler = 8 per day; 8-ounce cup = 16 per day

Day 1	Day 2	Day 3	Day 4	Day 5
Day 6	Day 7	Day 8	Day 9	Day 10
Day 11	Day 12	Day 13	Day 14	Day 15
Day 16	Day 17	Day 18	Day 19	Day 20
Day 21	Day 22	Day 23	Day 24	Day 25
Day 26	Day 27	Day 28	Day 29	Day 30

Sorry Cellie!

Living in a storage closet with another person is hard enough, and when you add the restroom into the equation, it's just a crazy situation we put ourselves in. To add to that, we've all had that cellmate (cellie) who is always using the restroom. Well, I was "that cellie" when I started the 30-Day H_2O Gallon Challenge. Every morning, I would fill my pitcher and start drinking. My cellmate, whose nickname was Rambo, hated the toilet flushing, but he put up with it because he knew I was on a weight-loss mission, and drinking lots of water was part of that. I constantly found myself saying, "Sorry, Cellie," when I flushed the toilet all through the day. He would tell me he didn't care, but I still felt bad.

Eight days into the challenge, I continued to down my half gallon/one pitcher before afternoon chow, but I only used the restroom twice. For the last seven days, it had been about eight or more times. I figured my body had adjusted to the new routine, and I thought that was cool in itself. I had changed my body!

My cellie was happier, too. Although he never admitted to being annoyed, I know he was. My advice to anyone is to let your cellie know; let your boss, your coworkers, and whoever else may be affected by your constant restroom usage that you are doing the 30-Day H_2O Gallon Challenge. Even better yet, get them to do it with you! I feel great and continue to drink at least one gallon of water each day.

– Jayden O.

"Some people are always grumbling that roses have thorns. I am thankful thorns have roses." – Alphonse Karr

How you look at the rose is not the same as anyone else does. Some see a flower; some see wedding bells. It's different for everyone. The same goes for your health journey. Making sure to keep your outlook positive will guarantee a positive experience.

CHAPTER FIVE

Prisoner's Nutrition Guide

Being incarcerated and having your meals scheduled for you can make it difficult to really know how many nutrients you are getting from each meal. Unless you work in the kitchen, and sometimes not even then, you can't simply look at the food label to see how much trans-fat or sodium you will ingest at dinner tonight. We will go over the areas of nutrition that affect us the most, and a few areas for when you get out, or you can share with your family.

Fat, calories, saturated fat, protein, cholesterol, calcium, carbohydrates, sugar, fiber, potassium, vitamin C and folic acid –these are the nutrients that keep your body working every day. Yes, the list is lengthy, but your body handles these easily. Even as you are dreaming, your body is directing these nutrients to their proper destinations. A plus is that you can get most of these nutrients from foods you already love and enjoy. Depending on the food, you will receive different nutrients. Certain foods, like cheese and meat, are very high in protein content. Dairy products such as milk have loads of calcium. If you are in need of fiber, vegetables and fruits work wonders because they are packed with fiber. You will also receive a healthy dose of vitamins from these foods. Simply by having a wide variety of foods, you will guarantee yourself an assortment of nutrients!

When it comes to certain nutrients such as carbohydrates, protein, potassium, fiber, calcium, vitamin C, and folic acid, your mission is to ingest the right amount each day for maximum health. If you're wondering about calories, those are easy; eat just the right amount to keep your body energized and running properly. But don't consume so many calories that you start to gain pounds.

This portion of the book is geared to teach you the different nutrients, how they each affect your body, and which ones you should seek out more than others for your individual needs. Our bodies are all different, but we can do this together. You know better than anyone what your body needs and already has. This section will simply point out what each nutrient does and if it applies to you. Make it a point to get more of it, and if not, cancel that nutrient!

Calories

Calories, such a filthy word to many of us. We can't get away from them. Other than water, all food and drink have calories, even if it's only one. Whether you are eating a carrot or a double fudge cake, you will ingest calories. Your body is a fine-tuned machine that uses calories, food, as energy. Calories are the fuel.

When the fuel you put in equals the energy output, your weight remains steady. If you take in more fuel than you need, your body will save it for the future. This means your weight goes up. Your body will store this excess fuel as fat wherever it decides to. Be it your thighs, backside, or arms, you know where your body stores this excess. The trick is to take in fewer calories than you need. This will force your body to burn up the fat that it stored for future use. Well, now is that future!

If you recognize this fat storage dialogue from the Carbohydrate Wean Section, you are on the right track. Good job! Calories come directly from carbohydrates, fats, and proteins. Fat has the highest calorie content out of all nutrients, nearly twice as much as carbohydrates and proteins. Two teaspoons of fat have approximately 80 calories, whereas two teaspoons of carbohydrates have approximately 38 calories.

Studies have shown time after time that when a person consumes fewer calories, weight loss occurs. Watch out for the "Health Foods" because calories are calories, no matter how they are labeled. If you eat too many of them, you will gain weight. It makes no difference if those calories are coming from pizza, cookies, cinnamon rolls, and soda pop or broccoli, bananas, eggs, and milk. Too many calories are not a good thing if you really want to lose weight. In order to lose weight, the secret is burning more fat by eating fewer calories.

Estimated Calorie Requirements

The chart below is a rough guide to how many calories a person needs each day. Find your age range and your activity level, and that is the number of calories you should shoot for if not less.

3,500 Calories

If you want to gain a pound, you must eat 3,500 calories. If you want to lose a pound, you must burn 3,500 calories. I know your goal is to lose a pound, so let's look at the numbers to reach this goal. Your body is going to do most of the work.

Take your weight and multiply it by 10.2. Using my weight as an example (at my heaviest of 276 pounds), multiplying 276 pounds by 10.2 equals 2,815.2 calories. Wow! This is the number of calories my body burns "at rest," meaning as I do absolutely nothing. If I am sleeping, watching TV, or reading a book, I will burn 2,815 calories! If my goal is to lose a pound (3,500 calories), I can subtract my at-rest total from my goal (3,500 - 2,815 = 685), which means that I only need to burn 685 more calories to reach 3,500 calories, thus losing a pound. I could do an intense workout, burning up 700 calories, and I would surpass my goal by 15 calories.

Does that sound too good to be true? Well, if you were fasting for the whole day, this is exactly how it would be, but if you are like most people, you are going to eat today, so the example above still stands, but eating calories is going to take away from your "at rest" calories. This means the 2,815 "at rest" calories still stands, but when you eat 800 calories at lunch you have to subtract those 800 calories at lunch you have to subtract those 800 calories from your 2,815 "at rest" calories: 2,815 − 800 = 2,015.

Now I'm much further away from reaching 3,500 calories. Instead of needing only 685 calories to reach 3,500 like before, now I need 3,500 - 2,015, or 1,485 calories to go! When I eat 1,000 calories at dinner, I must subtract that too: 2,015 − 1,000 = 1,015 calories. Now I am far from 3,500 calories. Any snacks I eat during the day must also be subtracted. If I eat a pack of crackers totaling 100 calories, I need to take my 1,015 and subtract 100 calories. Now I'm at 915. Here is some good news: exercise is the only way to increase your total towards 3,500.

Now that I'm at 915 calories toward 3,500, I go outside and do a workout session, burning 430 calories. I can add that to my calories burned for the day: 915 + 430 = 1,345 calories burned. That is the end of my day, and I start fresh tomorrow. At this pace, it will take me about three days to lose a pound, being that 1,345 x 3 days = 4,035 calories burned. My mission was 3,500 calories, but I burned 4,035 instead. This means I went over by 530, and I can put that towards my next 3,500 calories burned to lose another pound!

Here it is in a nutshell:

- Step 1: Multiply your body weight by 10.2.

  _____ x 10.2 = _____
  your body weight   total

- Step 2: Add up all the calories you ate for the day and subtract them from the above total:

  _____ - _____ = _____
  above total   calories eaten   total 2

- Step 3: Figure out how many calories you burned by exercise and *add* that to the total 2.

  _____ + _____ = _____
  total 2   calories burned by exercise   final total

- Step 4: That final total is what you have burned towards 3,500 calories, AKA 1 pound lost. Make sure not to go into the negative. If you go backwards in your numbers, going below zero after step 2, you are on your way to gaining a pound. Stop that immediately; cut your calorie intake to get out of the hole and follow the 4-step plan. It all happens one pound at a time, and this is a way to track this process.

  Try sending a note to your kitchen or food service department and ask for a calorie menu to help you figure out your intake. Use the charting table on the following page to help you keep track of how many calories you're burning every day.

Multiply your current weight by 10.2 to determine your calories burned at rest. This will remain the same until you have lost more than five pounds. It is good to reassess every month because as you lose weight, your body burns less.

Each day you burn more calories than you take in is a victory. Draw a star in the last column. Each time you reach 3,500 calories, you have lost a pound. Draw a line and start again.

DATE	BREAKFAST TIME			LUNCH TIME			DINNER TIME			CALORIES BURNED		TOTAL CALORIES		CALORIE DIFFERENCE		:) or ✐
	MEAL	SNK	EXER	MEAL	SNK	EXER	MEAL	SNK	EXER	REST	EXER	BURN	IN	DAILY	CUMU	
samp	500	100	100	400	300	-------	600	55	-------	1950	100	2050	1955	95	95	✐
samp	550	130	-------	450		-------	700		400	1950	400	2350	1830	520	615	✐

The "Cumu" (cumulative) column before the star is where you add your final total from step 3 every day until you reach 3,500 calories.

Fat

Well, if any nutrient has a bad reputation, it's fat. It is definitely an undeserved reputation because fat is so important to the body. Fat provides energy, supplies necessary fatty acids that the body can't make, insulates the body, protects vital organs, carries fat-soluble vitamins, and becomes part of cell membranes. And if that's not enough, fat makes food taste delicious.

Fat (which scientists call lipids) is an umbrella term for many similar substances. You get fat from the foods you consume, and your body is capable of making certain fats. Fatty acids make up strands of food fats. Try to think of fatty acids as strands of beads that are different colors, combinations, and numbers of beads, depending on their chemical makeup.

The three main fatty-acid types are saturated, polyunsaturated, and monounsaturated. Foods have combinations of all three, but we make the labels saturated (butter), polyunsaturated (corn oil), and monounsaturated (olive oil), in direct relation to the predominant fat in the food. Studies show that the type of fat you consume is possibly more important than the amount of fat you eat.

How Much Fat Should You Consume?

Health experts recommend that your daily fat consumption be 20-30% of your total calorie intake. An example is if you typically ingest 1,800 calories per day, you should have between 360-510 calories come from fat. Take your daily planned calories and multiply by .30 to find out what 30% equals, i.e.,

_____ x .30 = calories from fat you should eat.
(daily calories)

To be perfectly clear, although studies continue to prove that a moderate fat diet can be healthy, I am not promoting a high-fat diet or saying it is great for you. Keep your fat intake under 30% of your daily intake of calories. A neat trick is keeping your carbohydrates low and eating healthy fats such as meat and cheese. This will give your body a chance to burn those fats up right away. Now your body is a fat-burning zone and will immediately start burning fat recently stored in your body. Not only do you get to eat some tasty food, but you also get to supercharge your metabolism into burning stored fat.

Saturated Fat

I have read several expert studies that call out saturated fats as the enemy of dieters, mainly because saturated fats play a role in raising a person's blood cholesterol levels. Saturated fats are mainly found in meats, milk, cheese, and other animal foods. Coconut oil and palm oil also contain saturated fats. It is nearly impossible to eliminate saturated fats from your diet, but you don't have to; all you need to do is keep your saturated fats as low as possible. It's so simple, especially when it comes to food items, where you can have the option of low-fat. Just read the labels when you can, and if you are not sure, eat smaller portions.

What is the Right Amount of Saturated Fat to Eat?

Surprisingly, there has never been a specific recommendation made when it comes to saturated fat. What is most commonly said is to keep your saturated fat intake low. Well, that leads to the question, "How low do I go?" The National Cholesterol Education Program has suggested that about 7% of your daily calories come from saturated fat. Other organizations have recommended 10% or less. Using logic and realizing that we already consume 13-15% of our daily calories as saturated fat, any reduction, especially under 10% would give you the health benefits you are looking for.

Using our 1,800-calories-a-day example from earlier, let's go with 8% of your calories coming from saturated fats to keep it under 10%. You would multiply 1,800 by .08, which equals 144 calories of saturated fat per day. In other words, your daily calories times the percent of fat per day you're aiming for equals the total calories from saturated fat you can eat. To find percent: 4% = .04/ 5% = .05/ 6% = .06, etc., until you get to double digits (which we are trying to avoid), at which point it goes 10% = .10/ 11% = .11/ 12% = .12, etc. Remember, by lowering your total fat intake, you lower your saturated fat intake by default.

Cholesterol

Cholesterol is a waxy, white, fat-like substance that can be found in every single cell within your body. It is an insulator to your nerves and assists your skin cells in holding onto and retaining moisture. Cholesterol makes up a large part of your brain! Cholesterol is also a foundational building block that makes up testosterone, estrogen, cortisone, and even vitamin D. There is a downside to cholesterol; having too much in your blood is very unhealthy for anyone. Your body will dispose of the extra cholesterol on your artery walls, which typically makes them narrow, weakening blood flow all throughout your body. An interesting fact is that your body can actually make cholesterol!

As a matter of fact, the human body usually creates over two times the cholesterol that a person consumes through food!

You will take in cholesterol every time you digest meat, milk, poultry, eggs, fish, butter, and/or cheese. You will never ingest cholesterol if you digest fruits, vegetables, seeds, nuts, grains, and/or cereals like oats, anything from the earth basically.

What's the Right Amount of Cholesterol?

The average American male will eat about 350 milligrams (mg) of cholesterol per day. The average American woman will eat about 250 mg of cholesterol per day. The U.S. Government's National Cholesterol Education Program suggests a maximum of less than 200 mg of cholesterol per day, whether male or female. The American Heart Association recently recommended that a person limit their daily cholesterol intake to 300 mg or less. If you already have heart complications, the number drops to 200 mg per day.

Use your most recent blood test to figure out your daily cholesterol needs. When your LDL (low-density lipoproteins) or "bad" cholesterol levels are above the desired range, drop your daily cholesterol intake down to 200 mg per day. This will help your body regulate your cholesterol. Keep in mind that if it grew from the earth, it has zero cholesterol; if it comes from an animal, it has cholesterol.

Protein

Every single day, your body loses millions of cells. This happens for all sorts of reasons. Some cells are worn out, used all the way up, or cut off like one of your toenails. Because of this loss, you need a good source of quality protein to replenish the dead cells.

Protein can be found in every one of your cells, every tissue and substance within you, except bile and urine. Muscles, bones, teeth, skin, enzymes, and blood all contain high amounts of protein. The more active a body part is, the more protein it has; the less active tissues naturally contain less protein.

Amino acids are the small building blocks that make up protein. The body uses twenty amino acids to build various proteins. Combining two numbers can make a new number, just like 5-4-1 combined makes 541; the amino acids combine to make new proteins. Out of the twenty different amino acids, nine are essential. These nine are found in the food you eat and must be consumed by eating. As for the other eleven, your body will make those. Whenever you consume different foods, you get various combinations of proteins and amino acids. That is the main reason you should eat a variety of food if you want to get more protein.

Nearly all foods contain some level of protein, some more than others. Meat, for example, has much more protein than fruits. Vegetables, milk, grains, cheese, and beans all have a higher protein content than fruit.

When your body is stressed mentally or physically, you lose protein. Nitrogen is eliminated during times that you are heavily sweating, and protein is necessary to replace the nitrogen. When you deal with an injury, surgery, infection, fever, or even when you exercise, your body is in need of protein. A mental stress, such as a breakup, job loss, or prison sentencing, can cause protein loss.

How Much Protein Do I Need?

First, divide your weight in half. This number is the amount in grams of protein you should consume per day. For example, if you weigh 250 pounds, 250 divided by 2 is 125. Therefore, you should eat 125 grams (g) of protein per day. It's that simple, and you'll be shocked to see how easy this is to do. Chances are you've been eating more protein than you realize; just be consistent.

The Top 10 Protein Sources

- Poultry
- Beef
- Milk
- Yeast Bread
- Cheese
- Eggs
- Fish
- Fresh Pork
- Ham
- Pasta

I personally would stay away from pasta while you are working towards your weight-loss goals, but once you get down to where you want to be, it's nice to know that you can enjoy some pasta!

It's important to remember to stick to your eating plan along with everything else we've discussed, such as your water intake.

Carbohydrates

Remember to reread the Carbohydrate Wean System. Simple carbohydrates are foods that contain large amounts of sugars. Carbohydrates include starches and fiber within foods. All-natural plant foods are loaded with carbohydrates. Vegetables, fruits, grains, and beans all contain carbohydrates. Fruits tend to contain more sugar. Grains, vegetables, and beans have more starch. All of these contain fiber.

Your body's main source of energy is in the form of sugars and starches. As the food you eat begins to get digested, sugar begins to enter the bloodstream by turning itself into molecules and moving into cells. Once the sugar is there, it is burned for energy so your body can stay functional.

Starch molecules are complex. They are made up of lots of sugar molecules which are bound together as one. When your body is digesting sugar, the sugar moves very simply. When digesting starches, they have to be broken down slowly to make way for smaller sugar fragments, which can now be sent to the cells and burned for energy. The problem is, once you eat more carbohydrates than your body *needs*, the leftovers are stored as fat.

How do I Count Carbs?

In the not-so-distant past, we were told to eat as many carbohydrates as we pleased. As a matter of fact, most inmates get 60% or more of their weekly calories from carbohydrates. Today, after much scientific research, carbohydrates are the villain that is responsible for many health problems we face today. Obesity is the top health issue that stems from excessive carbohydrates. Obesity, in turn, has a wide array of health issues that come with it. This makes the answer to the question of how many carbohydrates you should be eating very important.

The National Academy of Sciences Recommended Dietary Allowances (RDA) for carbohydrates is 130 g per day. The Food and Drug Administration (FDA) has set the Daily Value (DV) for carbohydrates at 300 g per day for the typical American diet.

A good way to estimate your personal carbohydrate intake is by choosing the amount of carbohydrates you want to eat each day. Most food experts consider 100 grams of carbohydrates or less to be where the most weight loss results happen while keeping the body energized.

Choose foods that are higher in fiber and lower in sugar. There are carbohydrates in vegetables as well as cookies, but do you think they are stored as fat in the same way? Absolutely not! Vegetables are a complex carbohydrate, and cookies are a simple carbohydrate. Remember, simple carbs are foods that have lots of sugars, such as desserts, jelly, honey, syrup, and sweets.

Complex carbs are foods that contain lots of starch, such as vegetables, beans, whole grains, and cereals. They are also rich in vitamins, fiber, and minerals. Because complex carbs take longer to be broken down into sugar, you have a better chance of burning up those complex carbs first.

It should not come as a surprise that I am not a big fan of carbohydrates. I mean, I have a copyrighted program called the Carbohydrate Wean System, where you eliminate carbs from your life. Now that you are a bit more educated on the different kinds of carbohydrates there are, you can see that my main focus is the elimination of simple carbohydrates from your diet. While you are on your weight-loss journey, carbohydrates in their simple form are not your friends, and you need to pay extra close attention to what complex carbohydrates you are consuming. Once you get to where you'd like to be, you can start introducing more carbohydrates of any kind back into your diet. Until then, be very careful.

Sugar

Do you have a sweet tooth? I know I do! Anthropologists have theorized that our capability to taste the differences between bitter plants and sweet plants could have contributed to human survival over time, because bitter plants were typically poisonous, and sweet plants were edible and good!

In today's world, however, our lust for sweets is creating the obesity epidemic (see carbohydrate section). Obviously, we are allowing our sweet tooth to make our dietary decisions, while the foods containing the real nutrients are not chosen. In the United States, more soda pop is consumed than milk! While vegetables, fruits, cereals, milk, grains, and yogurt all contain sugar, these are natural sugars. Cookies, cakes, soda, jelly, ice cream, candy, syrup, and fruit drinks, on the other hand, are packed with *added* sugars.

How Much Sugar is Too Much Sugar?

The latest study shows 15-20% of Americans are not aware of any added sugars in their diets. Also, Americans currently consume nearly 25% of their daily calories from sugar. When sugar intake spikes, vitamin and mineral intake falls. All of us need to eat less sugar, but we have no guidance about the specific recommendation on how much to eat on a daily basis. The United States Dietary Reference Intake (DRI) suggests 25 25% of your daily calories be from added sugar at the maximum. Clearly, that number is too high, and people should eat much less than that. The World Health Organization (WHO) suggests limiting added sugars to less than 10% of your total calories.

Because there is no point-blank recommendation, you need to choose for yourself how much sugar to eat each day. My recommendation is to try to eat *no* sugar every day. It will make you feel so much better, and when you do "accidentally" eat a cookie, the impact won't be as bad. Choose natural sugars and stay away from added sugars. This will keep you steady on your weight-loss goals.

Tip: To find added sugars, read the label and see if you find any of the following, which are other terms for sugar.

- Brown Rice Syrup
- Beet Juice
- Barley Mart
- Honey
- Corn Syrup
- Cane Syrup

- Brown Sugar
- Maltodextrin
- Malt Syrup
- Invert Sugar
- Dextrose
- Molasses
- Maple Syrup
- Maple Sugar
- High Fructose Corn Syrup
- Fructose
- Cane Juice
- Sorghum
- Raw Sugar
- Turbinado Sugar
- Sucrose

As you can see, there are a lot of ways sugar is labeled and introduced to us. Take this seriously because, as you can see, the main topic of this book is how sugar is stored as fat. All of these are sugars and can be stored as fat. Be sure to double-check your labels and avoid added sugars.

Fiber

Fiber is a certain type of carbohydrate that your body cannot digest and offers no calories. Fiber is very important, though. The fiber in the foods we consume assists us in losing weight, relieving constipation, and protecting against colon cancer. Some studies even show that fiber reduces your risk for heart disease.

Do not start going super heavy on fiber-rich foods right away. Add fiber-rich foods into your diet slowly. Vegetables, fruits, oatmeal, bran, grains, berries, beans, and popcorn all contain fiber. It does take your body a while to adjust to the new nutrients passing through your digestive tract. Also, remember to drink lots of water because fiber is like a sponge, the way it soaks up water. Fiber not only helps you feel fuller, so you eat less, but fiber also helps your bowel movements pass more easily.

What's the Right Amount of Fiber?

Most inmates do not get enough fiber. On average, prisons offer 15 grams of fiber per day, which is significantly less than the recommended daily intake. Health experts have made a chart of recommendations for fiber consumption based on age and gender. Take a look:

Men's	Grams of Fiber Needed per Day
19-50 years old	38 g of fiber
50 years old and older	30 g of fiber

Women	
19-50 years old	25 g of fiber
50 years old and older	21 g of fiber
Pregnant/Postpartum	28 g of fiber

Look for foods that have 5 g of fiber or more per serving. These are high fiber foods. A good fiber source contains at least 2 g per serving.

Calcium

I remember growing up and being told that calcium would make my bones and teeth stronger. Now I am older and hear that calcium also helps protect from adult bone thinning, commonly known as osteoporosis. Calcium does all of that and so much more!

More than half of the calcium in the typical American diet comes from cheese, yogurt, milk, and ice cream. One glass of nonfat milk gives us more than 30% of our calcium for the day. Other good calcium sources are dark green leafy vegetables, oysters, clams, almonds, beans, and sardines.

A recent study shows the top 15 benefits of a steady calcium intake:

- Reduces the risk of kidney stones
- Helps blood clot
- Protects against infertility

- Helps nerves work properly
- Lowers the risk of tooth loss (periodontal disease)
- Allows the heart and muscles to perform optimally
- Promotes good cholesterol (HDL) in postmenopausal women
- Helps regulate high blood pressure
- May lower the risk of certain cancers
- Helps aid in weight loss
- Helps reduce certain complications during pregnancy
- Helps prevent midlife weight gain
- Relieves premenstrual syndrome (PMS)
- Helps strengthen bones
- Protects bones from thinning in adults (osteoporosis)

What is the Right Amount of Calcium for Me?

Here is a chart that goes for everyone, depending on age.

Age	Amount of Calcium Needed per Day
19-50 years old	1,000 mg of calcium
50 years old & older	1,200 mg of calcium

Sodium

As you can see, your body needs a certain amount of each nutrient daily to function properly, including the nutrients we heard are evil such as sugar, fat and carbohydrates. Well, nothing is different when it comes to sodium. Sodium regulates the fluid levels of your body's inside cells and outside cells. This oversees your blood pressure, blood volume and toxicity or acidity of your body. The flow of sodium in and out of cells makes way for other important materials to make the journey too. Sodium also helps your nerves communicate and conduct electricity which your body depends on second to second.

Sodium often gets a bad reputation because of its association with high blood pressure. It has been proven that in parts of the world where very little salt is used, high blood pressure simply isn't a concern compared to the U.S.A. and the U.S. Prison System, where salt is highly relied upon at every meal. If you already have high blood pressure, you can bring it down by eating less sodium. Even if you have regular blood pressure, eating less sodium is a wise choice. You will reduce your risk of kidney disease, heart attack, and stroke.

Eating less salt doesn't mean to just stop sprinkling salt over your food, although that is a great start. It means really reading the food labels and knowing what is sodium-heavy and what is not. Start by cutting down on foods with too much sodium and adding foods with less sodium.

How Much Sodium is the Right Amount?

Many prisons operate from the National Dietary Guidelines, which means most inmates eat an average of 3,500 milligrams (mg) of sodium per day! The recommended amount of sodium for adults is 1,500 mg, with older adults at around 1,000 mg per day. Actually, a person could do very well on 500 mg of sodium per day.

Here is a chart that shows the recommended sodium consumption for adults.

Age	Amount of Sodium Recommended per Day
19-50 years old	1,500 mg per day
50-70 years old	1,300 mg per day
70 years and older	1,200 mg per day

Fun Fact!

Table salt is in fact a combination of two minerals: chloride and sodium. Out of the 5,000 mg that are in a teaspoon of salt, 2,000 mg are sodium and 3,000 mg are chloride.

Sodium that is without chloride is found in monosodium glutamate (MSG). You can also find it in food additives such as sodium benzoate and sodium propionate, as well as in artificial sweeteners such as sodium saccharin. Medication also contains sodium citrate. Even in water, you will find the mineral sodium. It is safe to say that sodium in some form is everywhere. Let's just try not to consume so much into the body.

Potassium

Can you guess what the third-highest ranking mineral in your body is? If you guessed potassium, you are correct! You can find potassium in every single cell in your body. Nerves use it to help with firing off properly, and muscles use it to function. Your heart also uses potassium to relax. If you recall, this is the opposite of calcium, which helps the heart muscle contract. If you are dealing with high blood pressure, potassium can help regulate that. To strengthen your bones, eat fruits and vegetables that are rich in potassium. High potassium levels encourage your body to cling to calcium instead of disposing of it, which leads to stronger bones.

What is the Right Amount of Potassium?

There is so much potassium in the foods we eat that there is no Dietary Reference Intake (DRI) for potassium! The studies I have read have shown that about 1,800 mg per day is sufficient. No need to worry, the average American inmate consumes nearly 4,000 mg per day.

Folic Acid

The vitamin folic acid is a nutrient that everyone needs in order to guarantee that their cells develop correctly and reproduce. Since folic acid aids in the creation of all of the genetic material in your body, it is very important to get the right amount from the right sources. When a cell is forming, it needs folic acid to create the proper genetic material, the proper protein, and healthy red blood cells. If the right amount of folic acid isn't present in your body, red blood cells do not develop properly or last as long as other red blood cells.

Along with helping with fertility in both genders, folic acid helps to protect you from heart disease. It does this by lowering blood levels of homocysteine, a protein which is believed to be a contributor to heart issues.

You can get decent amounts of folic acid from foods like broccoli, peanuts, green leafy vegetables, orange juice, asparagus, and dried beans. A few fortified sources of folic acid are rice, enriched bread, pasta, and breakfast cereal.

What is the Right Amount of Folic Acid?

There is a daily DRI for folic acid. Here is a chart. Find your age and gender to figure out your daily needs.

Men	Amount of Folic Acid Recommended Daily
14 years old & older	400 micrograms (mcg)*
Women	
14 years old & older	400 mcg
Pregnant women	600 mcg
Breastfeeding women	500 mcg

*All labels show folic acid in micrograms, so don't worry about doing any crazy math, like turning milligrams into micrograms. Just aim for your number. You'll get it!

Vitamin C

Early ocean explorers often lost their lives due to a lack of vitamin C. While travelling the seas for months, even years at a time, with no source of fresh vegetables or fruits, many sailors died from scurvy. Vitamin C plays a critical role in the development of collagen, which is the connective tissue that keeps the structures of the body held together. Most tissues in your body contain collagen, but it's very prevalent in your brain, heart, lungs, eyes, and pancreas. Some would say these are some pretty important organs! The sailors we discussed earlier suffered from painful joint pain and bleeding gums because they had no way to make collagen. That is what led to their death.

Vitamin C is also in the antioxidant family. An antioxidant is a substance that acts as a shield to healthy cells. There are harmful substances known as "free radicals" that try to harm healthy cells. Antioxidants gather the free radicals and stop them in their tracks from causing damage to healthy cells, which could lead to cancer and heart disease. Air pollution, sun exposure, smoking, and chemical exposure are the main culprits of free radical production.

Vitamin E and other nutrients, such as folic acid, are protected by Vitamin C, which allows them to work more effectively throughout the entire body. The best sources of Vitamin C are citrus fruits (oranges, grapefruits), peppers, leafy green vegetables, potatoes, spinach, and cantaloupe.

What is the Right Amount of Vitamin C?

This chart contains the daily DRI for vitamin C intake. Find your gender and age to find your recommended intake.

Men	Amount of Vitamin C Recommended Daily
14 years old & older	90 mg
Women	
14 years old & older	75 mg
Pregnant women	85 mg
Breastfeeding women	120 mg

Dietary Guideline Basics

The dietary guidelines in the United States emphasize eating fewer calories, being more active, and making mindful food choices. In 1980, the United States Department of Agriculture (USDA), along with the Department of Health and Human Services (DHHS), initiated the dietary guidelines. These guidelines are to be passed on to the policymakers and promote the optimum eating schedule, stop diseases, and set the status quo for federal programs such as the National School Lunch Program. The dietary guidelines allow a baseline for all government agencies to have a common approach when it comes to delivering nutritional messages to their members, thus preventing mixed messages.

The law states that the DHHS and the USDA must elect a committee of certified experts to review all new scientific data and change the guidelines as new data appears. These committee members also convey the new information to normal people like us. By obeying these guidelines, you reduce your risk for obesity, diabetes, osteoporosis, heart disease, hypertension, and cancer.

Here are the latest dietary guidelines from DHHS & USDA:

- Balance your need for important nutrients with your daily caloric needs. When you reduce foods high in fats and sugars, you will free up calorie space for smarter food choices. You still take in the same number of calories, but the value of the food is improved. Reaching your daily nutrient needs has to go hand in hand with keeping your calorie intake in check, so that your weight doesn't go up.

- Balance food intake and physical activity to manage body weight. Whatever the amount of energy you use each day, it should be equal to the calories you eat; this way, you stay at the same weight or even lose weight, and your weight never goes up.

- Be physically active every day. Daily exercise or physical activity improves your well-being and health and will help you lose weight. People who exercise have a lower death rate, which I feel is a good thing.

Getting out of obesity or lowering your risk for obesity, diabetes, hypertension (high blood pressure), heart disease, and some cancers can all be accomplished with physical activity. Physical activity and exercise help manage anxiety and depression. A good goal to achieve is to aim for thirty minutes of physical activity per day, at least five or six days a week.

If weight loss is your goal, go for sixty minutes of physical activity at least four or five days a week. Switch your exercises from day-to-day or week to week. Variations include cardiovascular, stretching, and strength training, as well as combinations of the three known as cross-training, which will help you achieve your weight-loss goal.

The time involved may seem daunting for anyone beginning an exercise routine. A good way to achieve these minutes is to either get it done all at once or break a sixty-minute workout into four fifteen-minute workouts throughout the day. Doesn't that sound nice? We will go over different workout plans for later in this book to help you formulate a strategy. Even taking a brief walk, cleaning your cell, or pushing yourself a little harder at work can all contribute to your goal of reaching 30 or 60 minutes of physical activity.

According to the Dietary Guidelines, most Americans are not eating enough of the following nutrients:

- Vitamin A, found in liver, sweet potatoes, carrots, mango, spinach, cantaloupe, broccoli, watermelon, and prunes

- Vitamin C, found in orange juice, cantaloupe, strawberries, cauliflower, watermelon, spinach, pineapple, cabbage, and potatoes

- Vitamin E, found in sunflower seeds, almonds, peanuts, and margarine

- Calcium, found in cheese, milk, spinach, and salmon

- Potassium, found in bananas, orange juice, beans, potatoes, and tomato juice

- Magnesium, found in spinach, brown rice, peanut butter, and almonds

- Fiber, found in bran cereal, brown rice, fruits with skin, dried fruit, carrots, beans, green beans, and popcorn

It's important to remember these points:

- Eat a variety of nutrient-rich foods every day.

  Begin eating more whole fruits rather than drinking fruit juice. Eat more dark green vegetables such as broccoli. Orange vegetables such as sweet potatoes and carrots are great for you. Also, choose to eat more peas and beans, and eat at least 2-3 servings of low-fat dairy products per day.

- Choose your fats wisely.

  Choose a daily fat intake of 20-30% of your total caloric intake each day. Maintain your intake of cholesterol and saturated fat by lowering the number of animal fats, such as fatty meat, cheese, butter, bacon, sausage, and skin from poultry that you consume. Make sure to limit your saturated-fat intake to less than 10% of your daily caloric intake.

- Stay away from trans-fats.

  The main sources of trans-fats are crackers, cookies, pastries, cakes, deep-fried foods (French fries, fried chicken), and stick margarine. Trans-fats raise your cholesterol, lower HDL (good cholesterol), raise LDL (bad) cholesterol, and increase one's risk for heart disease.

- Choose your carbohydrates wisely.

  Sugars, starches, and fiber are extremely vital for a healthy diet. Vegetables, fruits, grains, beans, and milk are major sources of carbohydrates that are beneficial to your diet. Because carbohydrates are a major source of calories in most diets, it is very important that you are careful as to what type of carbohydrates you are taking in. The strategy to lose weight is to eat more nutrient-rich foods and limit your intake of sugars and added sugars. Your focus needs to be on fruits and vegetables, and more peas and beans.

- Eat less salt and more potassium.

  Lessen the amount of salt you take in, and you lessen your chances of high blood pressure. Eating foods rich in potassium helps you control high blood pressure and build stronger bones. People who have normal blood pressure results have a lower risk of kidney disease, heart disease, stroke, and congestive heart failure.

  Processed foods are higher in salt content than homemade meals. In addition to the good sources of potassium listed on the previous page, it can be found in cantaloupe and spinach.

All in all, being in prison prevents us from being able to fully know how many nutrients we are getting per meal, but the general idea is to eat healthier, and now you have an idea of how to navigate your chow hall a little bit better. For people in the real world, it is difficult for them to follow all the recommendations set forth by the Dietary Guidelines. Think of the Dietary Guidelines as just that, guidelines that will guide you to a healthier life, not a strict rule book.

CHAPTER SIX

How to Read Food Labels

When I first started my weight-loss journey, I thought I knew how to read food labels –it seemed so easy. I thought, "Hmm, I can eat these pretzels. They only have 200 calories and 250 mg of sodium. That really isn't too bad." Well, that was at first glance. Once I took the time to *read* the label, I noticed that the 200 calories and 250 mg were for each serving –a single serving is 22 pretzels. There are 5 servings per container, bag, or whatever is containing the item you are consuming: yes, 5 servings!

Let's take another look at this: 200 calories x 5 servings = 1,000 calories

250 mg of sodium x 5 servings = 1,250 mg of sodium

Oops! This was supposed to be a snack!

Let's *read* the following label:

Front	Back

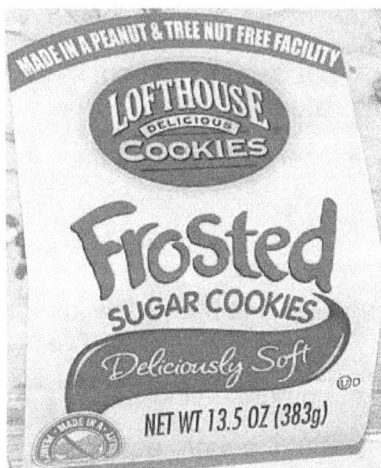

Nutrition Facts

Serving Size: 3 cookies
Servings per container: 10

Calories: 140
Fat: 15 grams
Saturated Fat: 8 grams
Cholesterol: 20 mg
Sodium: 310 mg
Carbohydrates: 50 grams
Sugars: 20 grams
Added Sugars: 10 grams
Protein: 2 grams
Fiber: 1 gram
Based on a 2,000-calorie diet

You see, all of the numbers for all of the nutrients, all the way down, are based on the serving size of 3 cookies. This means every time you eat 3 cookies, you must double whatever is on the label; if you eat all 10 servings, that equals 30 cookies. You have to multiply all these numbers by ten! That's 1,400 calories for starters.

Here are some of the tricks they use to confuse us. These are what manufacturers can claim on processed food labels:

Packaging Terms

Sugar

- Sugar Free: *Less than* 0.5 g per serving
- No-Added Sugar: No sugars or sugar-containing ingredients added *during processing*
- Reduced Sugar: *At least 25% less* sugar than the original food, meaning your favorite brand of chips might come out with a reduced-fat version. This new version needs to have at least 25% less per serving to meet the standard.

Fat

- Fat Free: *Less than* 0.5 g per serving
- Saturated Fat Free: *Less than* 0.5 g and trans-fatty acids per serving
- Low Fat: *3 g or less* per serving
- Low Saturated Fat: *1 g or less per serving* and not more than 15% of calories from saturated fat
- Reduced Fat: *At least 25% less* per serving than the original food

Fiber

- High Fiber: *5 g or more* per serving *and* meets low low-fat definition
- Good Source of Fiber: 2.5 g-4.9 g per serving
- More Fiber/Added Fiber: *At least 2.5 g more* per serving than the original food

Sodium

- Sodium Free: *Less than* 5 mg per serving

- Low Sodium: *140 mg or less* per serving

- Very Low Sodium: *35 mg or less* per serving

- Reduced Sodium/Less Sodium: *At least 25% less* per serving than the original food

Calories

- Calorie Free: *Less than 5 calories* per serving

- Low Calorie: *40 calories or less* per serving

- Reduced Calorie/Fewer Calories: *At least 25%* fewer calories than the original food

Cholesterol Free

- Cholesterol Free: *Less than* 2 mg *and* 2g or less of saturated fat per serving

- Low Cholesterol: *20 mg or less* of cholesterol *and* 2g or less of saturated fat per serving

- Reduced Cholesterol/Less Cholesterol: *At least 25% less* than the original food

Secondary Packaging Terms

The FDA permits food producers and advertisers to use certain words on their packaging that market to the public all of the health benefits they will receive by eating certain foods. If you see a product is *certified*, that means it has been evaluated by the USDA for class, grade, or characteristics of quality.

Why the Food and Drug Administrations are combined is a mystery to me, but here are some of the secondary packaging terms they allow.

Organic

- This product is produced by farmers who utilize environmentally friendly procedures to grow their livestock or plants. Before a product can officially be labeled organic, the farm and the farmer must be inspected by and receive approval from the USDA. Organic food must be grown without irradiation, sludge, sewage, synthetic fertilizers, illegal pesticides, and genetically modified organisms (GMOs).

Foods that contain all organic materials are allowed to print "100 percent certified organic" on the front of the package along with the USDA stamp. If a food only has 95% organic materials, it can print "organic" and still get the USDA stamp. If a product contains 70% organic material, they can say, "made with organic" on the front of the packaging, but no USDA stamp. Once a product goes under 70% organic, they cannot make *any* claims of organic anything on the front of the package, but can list "organic ingredients" on the side panel.

Natural

- The FDA has not set a clear definition for the term "natural" or any synonyms, but it can be used on packaging.

Free Range/Free Roaming

- Producers must prove that the poultry was allowed outside.

Fresh Poultry

- This includes whole poultry and cuts that have never been brought under 26 degrees F.

Gluten Free

- These products have a gluten limit of 20 parts per million.

Halal/Zabah Halal

- These products are produced in federally inspected meat packaging plants and handled in accordance with Islamic law and under Islamic authority.

Kosher

- This includes poultry and meat products prepared under rabbinical supervision.

No Antibiotics Added

- Hormones are strictly prohibited in the raising of pigs and poultry, so those products are not even allowed to make this claim. If a farmer can prove this to the USDA, the term might be allowed on packaging for beef.

No Antibiotics Added

- This claim can be added to a package of poultry and red meat if sufficient documentation is provided to the USDA proving the animals were raised without antibiotics.

As you can see, the farmers and the government agencies sent to police the farmers are a little shady. That is why it is good to understand food labels and how to read them.

Thank You Label!

All my boys were buying whey protein for almost 20 bucks a bag. All I could afford was peanuts, which I was told were a "great source of protein" on the front of the bag. The label on the protein bags said one scoop was 20 grams of protein; the label on my 30-cent peanuts said 11 grams of protein. I was bummed that my friends were getting about double the protein because I was poor.

I'll never forget the day that I was complaining to a guy (the author of this book) on the yard about my dilemma. He told me I was highly mistaken, and I needed to go back and read the label. I told him I had, and I knew what I was talking about. I'm not stupid! He calmly said, "Just look at the serving size and servings per container when you go back to your unit."

When I did, my mind was blown! The serving size was ⅓ of the bag, and there were 3 servings per container. Three servings in one bag of peanuts –that meant I could multiply 11 grams of protein by 3 servings. There were actually 33 grams of protein in each tiny bag of peanuts! I was getting more protein than all of my friends, and I didn't even know it, a lot more! All that protein for a fraction of what they were paying.

I've gotten pretty good at it now. Not all label readings give you an advantage like that, but knowing the rules of label reading can give you a head start on your goals and a leg up on the competition.

This experience also made me think about other times in my life when I thought I was lacking, but in reality, I was way ahead of the game. Well, I know how to read labels now. Don't get caught slipping like I did. Read the label!

– Josiah R.

CHAPTER SEVEN
Vitamin & Mineral Guide

Vitamins

Vitamin A

- Function: Promotes healthy eyesight, assists in the skin's ability to resist infection
- Sources: Liver, sweet potatoes, carrots, kale, cantaloupe, broccoli, fortified milk

Vitamin B_1/Thiamine

- Function: Vital to carbohydrate metabolism and nervous system health
- Sources: Eggs, enriched bread and flour, seeds, nuts, whole grains

Vitamin B_2/Riboflavin

- Function: Protects the eyes, mouth, skin, and mucous membranes; extremely essential to growth, metabolism, and red cell production
- Sources: Yeast, organ meats, almonds, mushrooms, whole grains, green leafy vegetables

Vitamin B_6/Pyridoxine

- Function: Very important in the regulation of the central nervous system and the metabolism of protein
- Sources: Bananas, whole grains, meat, avocados, fish, nuts

Vitamin B$_{12}$/Cobalamin

- Function: Necessary in forming red blood cells
- Sources: Poultry, meat, dairy products, eggs

Niacin

- Function: Maintains the health of the skin, the digestive system, and nerves
- Sources: Eggs, poultry, fish, nuts

Folic Acid

- Function: Required for new cells to form, grow, and reproduce, and for chemical reactions in the body's cells
- Sources: Leafy green vegetables, fruits, nuts, peas, cereals, dried beans

Other B Vitamins include biotin and pantothenic acid.

Vitamin C

- Function: Maintains collagen (a protein necessary for the formation of ligaments, skin, and bones
- Sources: Citrus fruits, broccoli, cantaloupe, tomatoes, potatoes, cabbage, sweet potatoes

Vitamin D

- Function: Essential to bone development
- Sources: Sunlight, milk products, oysters, tuna, sardines

Vitamin E

- Function: Assists in protecting red blood cells
- Sources: Eggs, peanuts, whole grains, green leafy vegetables

Vitamin K

- Function: Essential for the formation of prothrombin (allows blood to clot)
- Sources: Tomatoes and green leafy vegetables

Minerals

Calcium

- Function: Works together with phosphorus to build and maintain teeth and bones
- Sources: Green leafy vegetables, dairy

Phosphorus

- Function: Formation of teeth and bones, does more than any other mineral by showing up in every chemical reaction in the body
- Sources: Meats, cheese, milk, fish, and poultry

Iron

- Function: Necessary for the formation of good myoglobin (a safety supply of oxygen) for muscle tissue and hemoglobin, which transports oxygen throughout the bloodstream
- Sources: Beans, lean meats, green leafy vegetables, and whole grains

Other minerals include chloride, chromium, cobalt, copper, fluoride, iodine, magnesium, manganese, molybdenum, potassium, selenium, sodium, sulfur, and zinc.

"The best preparation for work is not thinking about or studying for work: It is work."
– William Weld

Putting the hammer to the nail is the best way to learn how to use it. It is understood that some people are visual learners, some are hands-on learners, and some are auditory (audio) learners, where they can just hear how to do something, and they can do it. The thing is that each type of learner has to eventually go and do the work; that's where the real learning takes place.

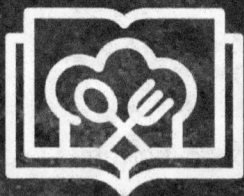

PART 2:
Cookbook & Meal Guide

*"We don't know who we are
until we see what we can do."*
– Martha Grimes

Sometimes, when I think I've been through it all and I know exactly how to handle any situation that comes my way, life throws a curveball and forces me to rethink everything I thought I knew. Going through a new situation will really show you who you are. I learned that I have way more self-control than I thought I had. That is huge because it ties directly into the way I eat and what I eat.

Once I saw that I was able to do it, I found out that the same self-control can be used in other aspects of my life. You really can change your entire life by learning what you are capable of during stressful or challenging situations. Today is the best day to start.

CHAPTER ONE

Main Dishes

Venezuelan Rice

Ingredients:
> ¼ bag of instant brown rice*
> 1 tablespoon soy sauce
> 1 pack of ranch dressing (low-fat or regular)
> 5 saltine crackers
> Unlimited jalapenos (optional)
> 1/4 teaspoon garlic powder
> Water
> 1 small pot and lid, 1 bowl, 1 cup, spoon

Instructions:
1. Pour rice into a bowl. Sprinkle garlic powder over the rice.
2. In a cup, put soy sauce, ranch dressing, and jalapenos together and stir.
3. Fill a small pot with the same amount of water as the rice being cooked. Heat the water to a boil.
4. Mix the rice in the water and reduce the heat to a simmer for 5 minutes with the lid on the pot. Remove from heat and let stand for 5 minutes, or until all the water is soaked up by the rice.
5. Uncover and pour in your Venezuelan sauce and mix until all is blended.
6. Crumble 5 or fewer saltine crackers on top of your meal and enjoy!

*If the rice being used is a different kind, follow the directions on the package.

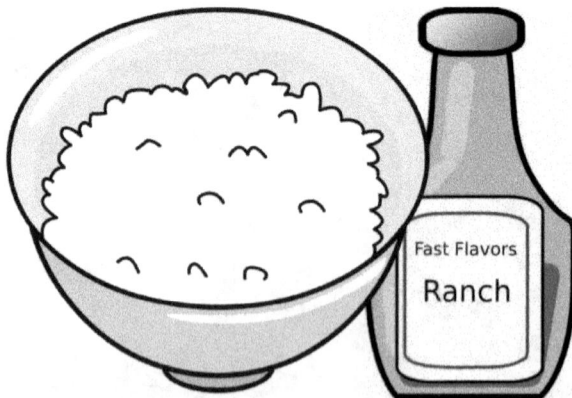

Mack Stack

Ingredients:

> 1/4 bag of instant brown rice
> 1 bag of pork rinds
> 1 pickle
> 1 pouch of mackerel (Jack Mack)
> 1 bag plain corn chips
> 1 squeeze cheese, single serve
> 1 sweeteners
> 1 packet of hot sauce
> Water
> 1 small pot and lid, 1 pitcher, 1 bowl, 1 spoon

Instructions:

1. In a pitcher, fill halfway with hot water and put the unopened mackerel pack in.
2. Fill a small pot with the same amount of water as the rice being cooked. Heat the water to a boil.
3. Mix the rice in the water and reduce the heat to a simmer for 5 minutes with the lid on the pot. Remove from heat and let stand for 5 minutes until all the water is soaked up by the rice, or cook according to the directions on the package.
4. Put the brown rice into the bowl.
5. Crush pork rinds inside the bag they come in. Put in the sweetener and hot sauce.
6. Shake the pork rind bag to mix it all together. Place to the side for later.
7. Use a spoon to pat down the rice and squirt cheese on top.

8. Take the mackerel package out of the water. Open and drain. Put on top of the bowl of rice.
9. Pour the pork rind mix evenly over the mackerel topping.
10. Crush up the corn chips and sprinkle over the pork rind mix.
11. Slice up the pickle to decorate the top of the bowl.

Enjoy!

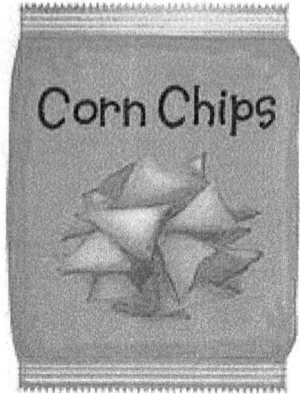

Vienna Rice

Ingredients:
>1/4 bag of instant brown rice
>1 can of Vienna chicken sausages (or any chicken)
>1 bag of pork rinds
>Unlimited jalapenos (optional)
>1 teaspoon garlic powder
>Water
>1 small pot and lid, 1 bowl, 1 spoon

Instructions:
1. Pour rice into a bowl, sprinkle garlic powder on top, and stir.
2. Fill a small pot with the same amount of water as the rice being cooked. Heat the water to a boil.
3. Mix the rice in the water and reduce the heat to a simmer for 5 minutes with the lid on the pot. Remove from heat and let stand for 5 minutes until all the water is soaked up by the rice, or cook according to the directions on the package.
4. While waiting, cut up Vienna chicken and add jalapenos into the chicken, pouring in jalapeno juice for more spice and flavor.
5. Crush pork rinds in the bag they come in. Add chicken and jalapenos and shake.
6. Uncover rice and pour in your pork rind/Vienna mix.

Combine all ingredients and enjoy!

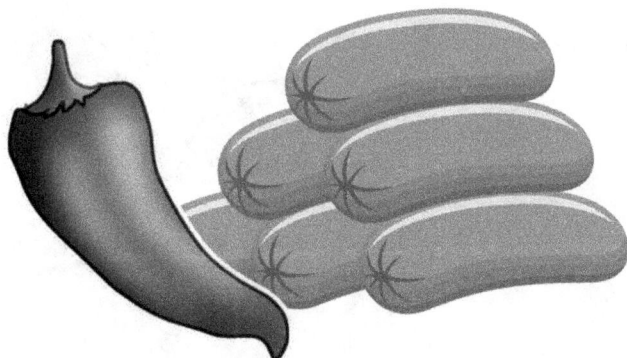

Peppered Rice

Ingredients:
1/4 bag of instant brown rice
Unlimited jalapenos (optional)
1 pack of ranch dressing
Black pepper to taste
Hot sauce
Water
1 small pot and lid, 1 bowl, 1 spoon

Instructions:
1. Fill a small pot with the same amount of water as the rice being cooked. Heat the water to a boil.
2. Mix the rice in the water and reduce the heat to a simmer for 5 minutes with the lid on the pot. Remove from heat and let stand for 5 minutes until all the water is soaked up by the rice, or cook according to the directions on the package.
3. Add pepper and stir, then cover with ranch dressing.
4. Lightly drizzle the hot sauce on top of the rice for flavor and decoration.
5. Eat up!

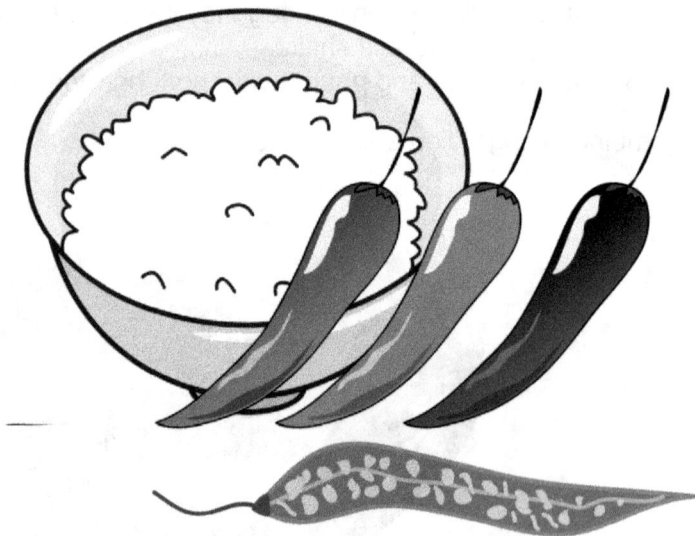

Pickled Rice

Ingredients:
> 1/4 bag of instant brown rice
> 1 teaspoon (tsp.) garlic powder
> 2 teaspoons of pickle juice
> 1 small pot and lid, 1 bowl, 1 spoon

Instructions:
1. Fill a small pot with the same amount of water as the rice being cooked. Heat the water to a boil.
2. Mix the rice and garlic in the water and reduce the heat to a simmer for 5 minutes with the lid on the pot. Remove from heat and let stand for 5 minutes until all the water is soaked up by the rice, or cook according to the directions on the package.
3. When the rice is done, pour in the pickle juice. So good!

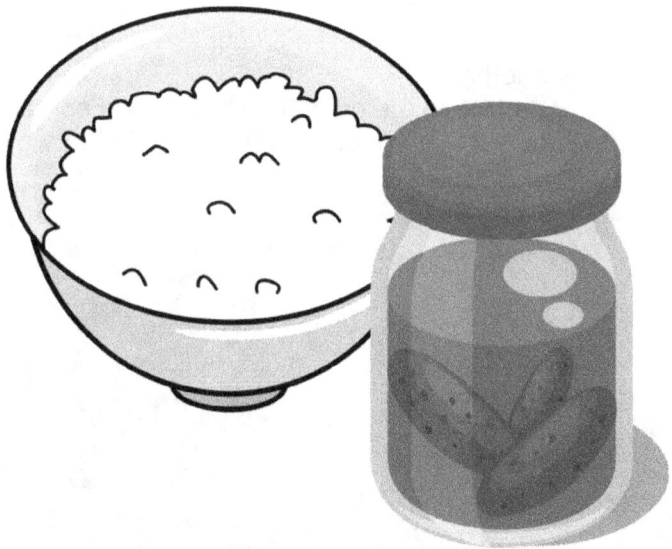

BOB (Ballin' on a Budget) Chicken Bowl

Ingredients:

¼ bag of instant brown rice
1 chicken stick or pouch (any chicken)
1 cheese squeeze single
Tapatio or any hot sauce
Water
1 small pot and lid, 1 bowl, 1 spoon

Instructions:

1. Fill a small pot with the same amount of water as the rice being cooked. Heat the water to a boil.
2. Mix the rice and hot sauce in the water and reduce the heat to a simmer for 5 minutes with the lid on the pot. Remove from heat and let stand for 5 minutes until all the water is soaked up by the rice, or cook according to the directions on the package. The rice should be slightly red.
3. While rice is cooking, cut up the chicken into smaller pieces. Set aside.
4. When rice is done, squirt cheese over rice and spread smoothly.
5. Put chicken on top of the cheese and spread evenly.
6. Leave it like it is or stir it together. Either way, it works and is tasty!

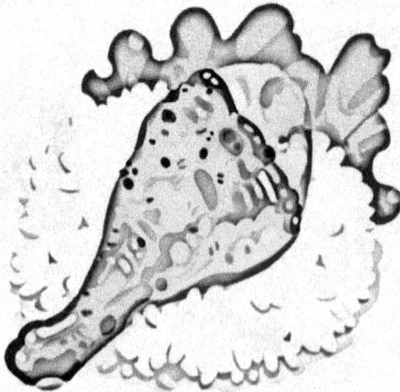

Orange Rice

Ingredients:
 1/4 bag of instant brown rice
 1 chicken pouch (shredded or chunked)
 1 orange Crystal Light (any brand)
 Unlimited jalapenos (optional)
 Water
 1 small pot and lid, 1 bowl, 1 spoon

Instructions:
 1. Fill a small pot with the same amount of water as the rice being cooked. Heat the water to a boil.
 2. Mix the rice in the water and reduce the heat to a simmer for 5 minutes with the lid on the pot. Remove from heat and let stand for 5 minutes until all the water is soaked up by the rice, or cook according to the directions on the package.
 3. Open the chicken pouch carefully across the top. Pour in half of the orange Crystal Light and gently massage the pouch to allow the drink mix to spread over all of the chicken.
 4. When the rice is done cooking, take off the lid and pour the other half of the orange Crystal Light over the rice and stir.
 5. Add jalapenos on top for flavor and decoration. Enjoy!

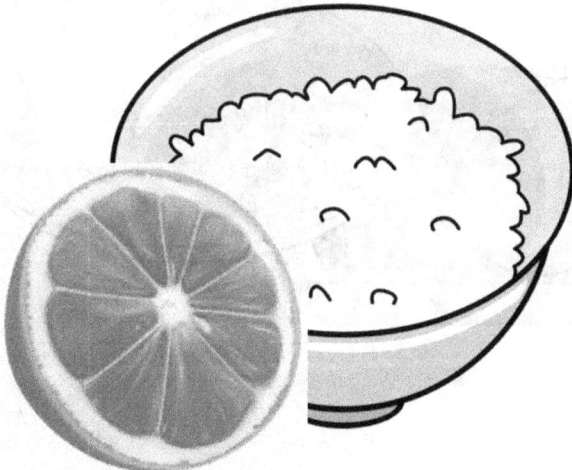

Mack Chicken Combo

Ingredients:
> 1 pack Jack Mack or any mackerel
> 1 pack of chicken (shredded or chunked)
> 2 cream cheese, single serving size
> 1 small bag of tortilla chips
> 2 bowls, 1 spoon

Instructions:
1. Cut up the mackerel in a bowl until no longer chunky.
2. Slightly open the chip bag to allow air to escape, then crush the chips into powder.
3. Dump powder over mackerel and stir until combined. Top with a lid and set aside.
4. In your second bowl, cut up the chicken and add all the cream cheese to the chicken.
5. Mix together until combined.
6. Now combine your first bowl with the second and mix until it all becomes one.
7. Try to eat it slowly … it will be hard!

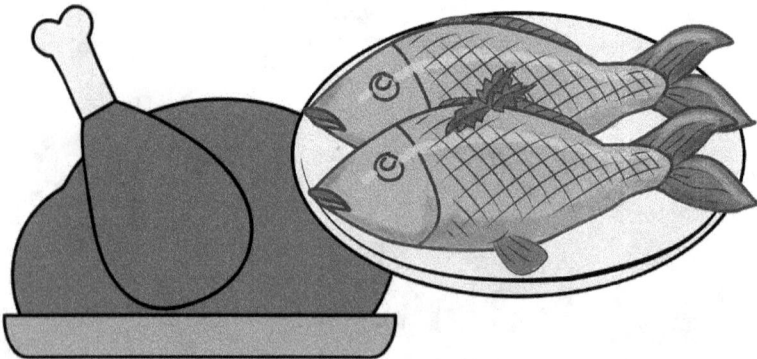

Chicken Fried Rice Bowl

Ingredients:
¼ bag of instant brown rice
4 spoonfuls of instant refried beans*
1 packet of chicken (shredded or chunked)
Unlimited jalapenos
1 cheese squeeze, single size
Water
2 small pots with lids, 1 bowl, 1 spoon

Instructions:
1. Fill a small pot with the same amount of water as the rice being cooked. Heat the water to a boil.
2. Mix the rice and jalapenos in the water and reduce the heat to a simmer for 5 minutes with the lid on the pot. Remove from heat and let stand for 5 minutes until all the water is soaked up by the rice, or cook according to the directions on the package.
3. In the other pot, put water (the same amount as the refried beans) and bring to a boil.
4. Put in the chicken and beans, turning it down to a simmer and covering the pot.
5. Stir it occasionally for 5 minutes. Let stand 5 minutes.
6. Combine the rice with the chicken mixture in the bowl, mixing well.
7. Squirt cheese on top and spread evenly. Dig in!

*If the refried beans being used are not instant, prepare according to package directions.

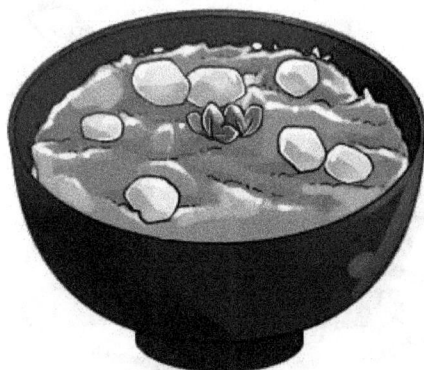

The Dippin' Chicken

Ingredients:
>1 package chicken (shredded or chunked)
>1/4 bag of instant brown rice
>1 pickle
>4 corn tortillas
>2 squeeze cheese, single serve
>Onion powder to taste
>Salsa
>1 small pot and lid, 2 bowls, 1 spoon

Instructions:
1. Fill a small pot with the same amount of water as the rice being cooked. Heat the water to a boil.
2. Mix the rice in the water and reduce the heat to a simmer for 5 minutes with the lid on the pot. Remove from heat and let stand for 5 minutes until all the water is soaked up by the rice, or cook according to the directions on the package.
3. In the first bowl, dump the chicken, sprinkling the onion powder on top.
4. Cut up the pickle into smaller chunks and combine with the chicken in the bowl.
5. Add salsa to that bowl and mix it all together.
6. In the second bowl, pour in the cooked brown rice, mixing it with the chicken.
7. Carefully scoop your chicken and rice mixture into the tortillas.
8. Squirt half of the squeeze cheese over each filled tortilla. You will love it!

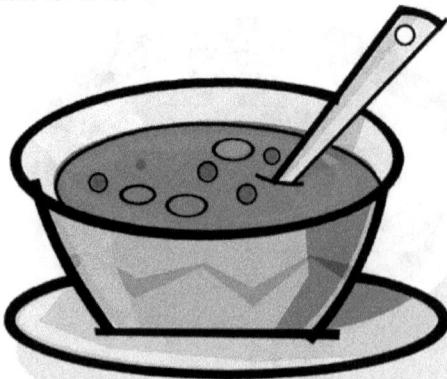

Lemon Pepper Chicken

Ingredients:
> 1/4 bag of instant brown rice
> 1 packet of chicken (shredded or chunked)
> 1 bag of pork rinds, crushed
> ½ tsp. black pepper
> ½ lemon Crystal Light, any brand
> 2 bowls, 1 spoon

Instructions:
1. Fill a small pot with the same amount of water as the rice being cooked. Heat the water to a boil.
2. Mix the rice in the water and reduce the heat to a simmer for 5 minutes with the lid on the pot. Remove from heat and let stand for 5 minutes until all the water is soaked up by the rice, or cook according to the directions on the package.
3. In a bowl, add crushed pork rinds, chicken, and pepper. Mix together.
4. When the chicken, rinds, and pepper are blended, sprinkle lemon Crystal Light over the top and fold in.
5. Put the rice in the other bowl and combine all ingredients. Mmm!

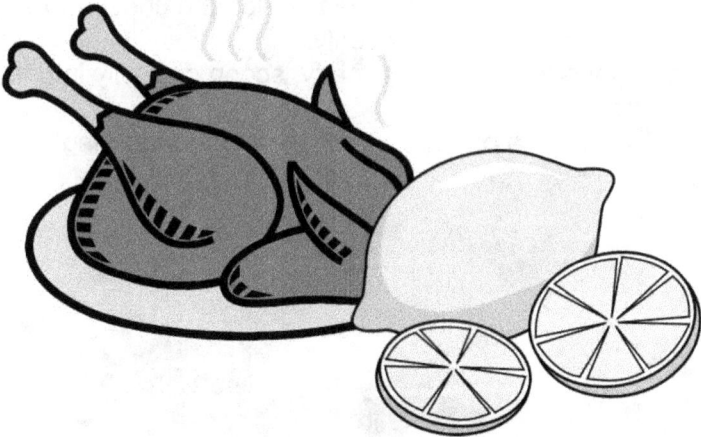

Brunch Burritos

Ingredients:
4 corn tortillas
2 Eggs, real or powdered
¼ bag of instant refried beans*
2 squeeze cheese, single serving
Salsa/peppers
Water
1 small pan and lid, 2 bowls, 1 spoon

Instructions:
1. If using real eggs, boil them by covering them with cold water, heating to medium for 1 minute to keep the shells from bursting (if they do burst, they will still work), then on high until they start to boil. Boil for 3 minutes, then turn off the heat source, leaving them there for 10 minutes. Pour out the water and put them into a bowl of cold water to peel.
2. Once peeled, smash them up until crumbly. If using powdered eggs, cook them according to package directions. Once they are ready, cover them with a lid and set aside.
3. Using the hot water from the eggs, heat again to a boil, using equal amounts of water and refried beans. Turn down the heat and simmer 5 minutes. Let it stand for 5 minutes. Or prepare according to package directions.
4. While waiting on the beans, add the cheese to each corn tortilla and spread evenly.
5. Once the beans are ready, scoop carefully into the tortillas.
6. Add salsa or peppers for zest. Good Morning!

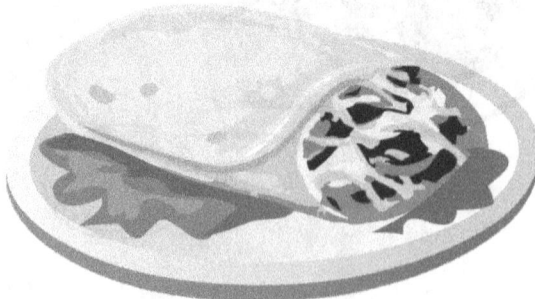

Cheesy Chicken Tacos

Ingredients:
> ¼ bag of refried beans
> ¼ bag of instant brown rice
> 1 packet of chicken (shredded or chunked)
> 1/4 cheese block, any kind
> 2 squeeze cheese, single serving
> Unlimited jalapenos
> 4 corn tortillas
> Water
> 1 small pot and lid, 2 bowls, 1 spoon

Instructions:
1. In the pot, put equal amounts of water as the rice and beans. Bring to a boil and add the rice and beans. Simmer for 5 minutes covered, then let stand for 5 minutes, or according to package directions if other than instant rice and beans are used.
2. In a bowl, dump in the chicken packet.
3. Cut up the cheese bar and add it to the chicken.
4. Cut up jalapenos and add them to the chicken and cheese. Set aside.
5. After the rice and beans are cooked, combine them with the ingredients from the second bowl, and stir together.
6. Squirt half a cheese squeeze onto each corn tortilla and spread evenly.
7. Carefully scoop your chicken mix into the tortillas. Yum! Yum!

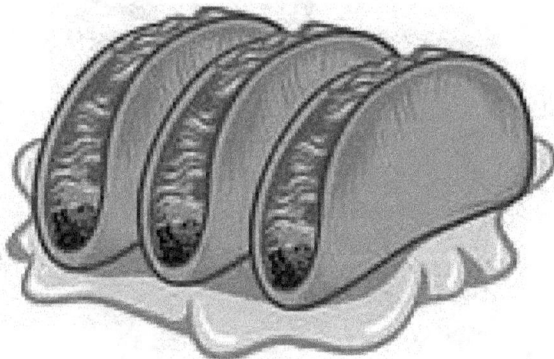

Blazin' Tuna Tacos

Ingredients:
1 pouch of tuna
4 corn tortillas
Unlimited jalapenos
1 hot pickle
4 squeeze cheeses, single size
Water
1 bowl, 1 spoon, 1 sealable plastic bag, 1 pitcher or hot pot

Instructions:
1. In your bowl, add tuna, cut up the pickle and jalapenos, and mix together.
2. Squirt half a cheese squeeze on each tortilla.
3. Carefully scoop tuna mix into each tortilla.
4. Wrap tortillas in an airtight plastic bag and place in a pitcher of hot water or a hot pot.
5. After 20 minutes, remove your wrapped tacos, unwrap, and eat. Tasty!

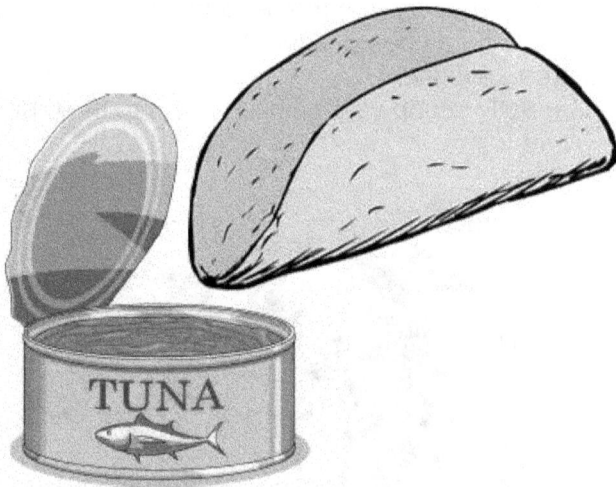

Speedy Chicken Bowl

Ingredients:
>1 package of chicken
>¼ bag of instant brown rice
>½ tsp. of garlic powder
>1 cheese squeeze, single size
>2 corn tortillas
>1 small pot and lid, 1 bowl, 1 spoon

Instructions:
1. Fill a small pot with the same amount of water as the rice being cooked. Heat the water to a boil.
2. Mix the rice and garlic in the water and reduce the heat to a simmer for 5 minutes with the lid on the pot. Remove from heat and let stand for 5 minutes until all the water is soaked up by the rice, or cook according to the directions on the package.
3. In a bowl, place 1 tortilla down so that the tortilla edges go up the sides.
4. Top the tortilla with the pack of chicken.
5. When rice is cooked, dump it on top of the tortilla and chicken in the bowl.
6. Place the second tortilla on top of the rice and carefully press down.
7. Squirt the cheese on top of the tortilla and spread evenly. Enjoy!

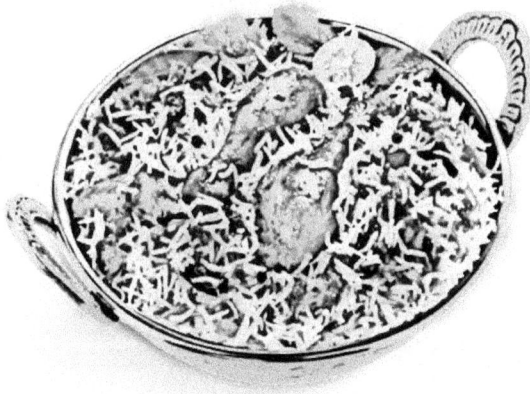

Southwest Poultry Wraps

Ingredients:
- 1 packet of chicken (shredded or chunked)
- ½ tsp. of garlic powder
- 1 single packet of ranch dressing
- 2 squeeze cheeses, single size
- Unlimited jalapenos
- 4 corn tortillas
- Hot sauce/salsa
- 1 bowl, 1 spoon

Instructions:
1. In your bowl, dump the entire packet of chicken, garlic powder, ranch dressing, cut-up jalapenos, and salsa. Mix all of the ingredients together thoroughly.
2. Squirt half of a cheese squeeze on each tortilla.

Carefully scoop the poultry mix from your bowl into the tortillas. Yee haw!

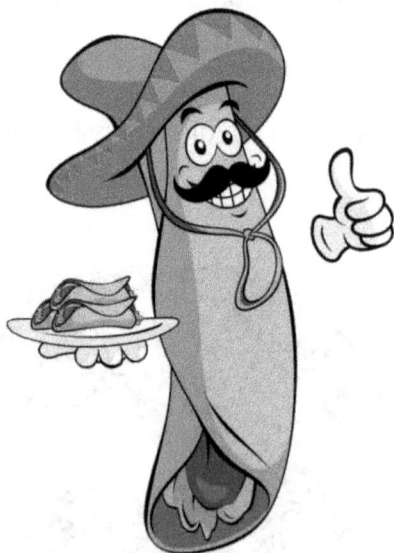

Chili Booms

Ingredients:

2 corn tortillas
1 package of chili (cooked or dry; if dry, cook according to instructions below)
Unlimited jalapenos
1 squeeze cheese, single size
¼ bag of instant refried beans
1 meat stick of your choice
Water
1 or 2 small pots and lids if cooking dry chili, 1 bowls, 1 spoon

Instructions:

1. In the pot, put an equal amount of water as the beans being used. Bring to a boil and add the beans. If instant beans, simmer for 5 minutes and set aside for 5 minutes. (If using a different type of beans, cook according to directions.)
2. If cooking dry chili, put it in the second pot, cover with water, and cook for 20 minutes or according to directions.
3. In a bowl, place one tortilla down.
4. Cut up the meat while waiting for the beans to cook.
5. When the beans are done, pour all the beans on top of the tortilla.
6. Place the second tortilla on top of the beans.
7. Squirt cheese on top of the tortilla, spreading evenly using a spoon.
8. Pour chili over the cheese and spread evenly using a spoon.
9. Add jalapenos and meat on top of the chili. Oh yeah!

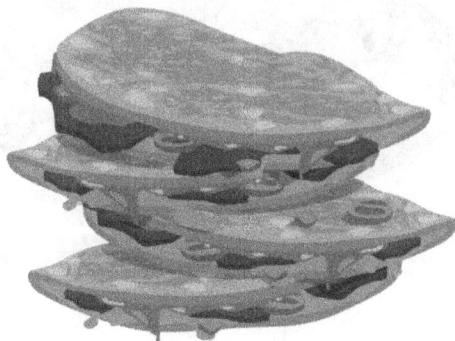

The BOB Boom

Ingredients:
>2 corn tortillas
>¼ bag of instant refried beans
>Unlimited jalapenos
>1 squeeze cheese, single serving
>Water
>1 small pot and lid, 1 bowl, 1 spoon

Instructions:
1. In the pot, measure an equal amount of water for the refried beans being used. Bring to a boil. Reduce to a simmer, covering with a lid, and let cook for 5 minutes. Remove from heat and let stand for 5 minutes, or prepare according to directions if the beans are not instant.
2. In the bowl, place one tortilla down.
3. When the beans are done, pour the beans on top of the tortilla in the bowl.
4. Place the second tortilla on top of the beans.
5. Squirt the cheese over the tortilla and spread evenly with a spoon. Dig in and enjoy.

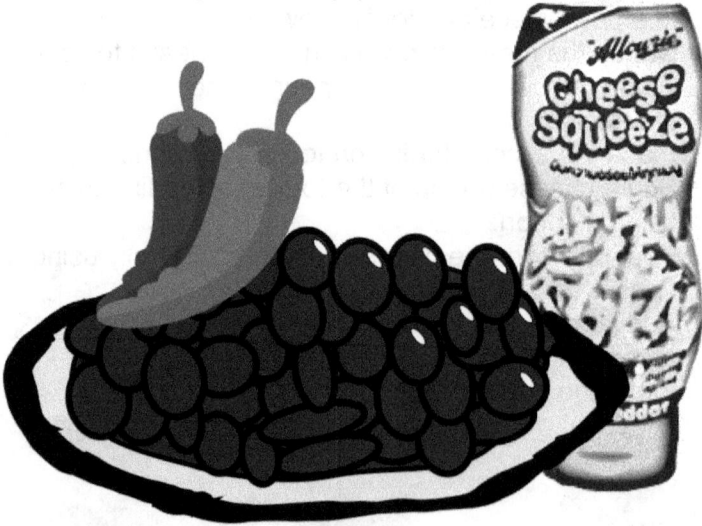

Tuna Booms

Ingredients:
>2 corn tortillas
>¼ bag of instant refried beans
>1 pouch of tuna fish
>1 squeeze cheese, single serving
>Water
>1 small pot and lid, 1 bowl, 1 spoon

Instructions:
1. In the pot, measure an equal amount of water for the refried beans being used. Bring to a boil. Reduce to a simmer, covering with a lid, and let cook for 5 minutes. Remove from heat and let stand for 5 minutes, or prepare according to directions if the beans are not instant.
2. In the bowl, place one tortilla down.
3. When the beans are done, pour them on top of the tortilla in the bowl.
4. Place the second tortilla on top of the beans.
5. Squirt the cheese over the tortilla and spread evenly with a spoon.
6. Open the tuna pouch and carefully drain the water out of the pouch. Dump tuna on top of the cheese. Eat up!

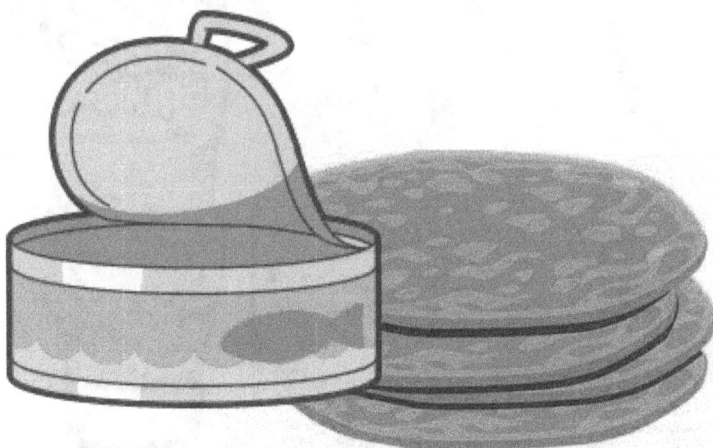

Jack Mack Booms

Ingredients:
>2 corn tortillas
>¼ bag of instant refried beans
>1 pouch of mackerel, any brand
>2 heaping scoops of instant brown rice
>1 squeeze cheese, single serving
>Water
>1 small pot and lid, 1 bowl, 1 spoon

Instructions:
1. In the pot, put equal amounts of water as the rice and beans. Bring to a boil and add the rice and beans. Simmer for 5 minutes covered, then let stand for 5 minutes, or according to package directions if other than instant rice and beans are used.
2. In the bowl, place 1 tortilla down.
3. When beans and rice are done cooking, pour them on top of the tortilla in the bowl.
4. Place the second tortilla on top of the beans and rice.
5. Squirt cheese on top of the tortilla.
6. Dump mackerel on top of the cheese. Try not to lick the bowl when it's done.

7.

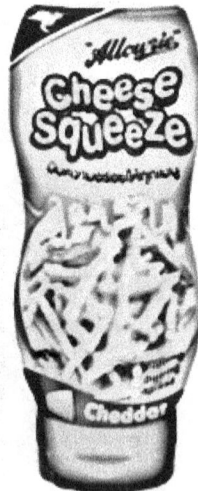

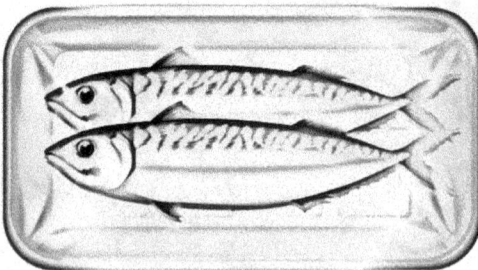

Sardine Booms

Ingredients:
> 2 corn tortillas
> ¼ bag of refried beans
> 1 pouch of sardines, any brand
> Unlimited jalapenos
> 1 squeeze cheese, single serving
> Water
> 1 small pot and lid, 1 bowl, 1 spoon

Instructions:
1. In the pot, put an equal amount of water as the beans. Bring to a boil and add the beans. Simmer for 5 minutes covered, then let stand for 5 minutes, or according to package directions if other than instant beans are used.
2. In the bowl, place one tortilla down.
3. When the beans are done, pour them on top of the tortilla in the bowl.
4. Place the second tortilla on top of the beans.
5. Squirt cheese on top of the tortilla, spreading evenly with a spoon.
6. Pump the ingredients from the sardine pouch on top of the cheese. Spread evenly with a spoon.
7. Place the jalapenos on top of the sardines and enjoy.

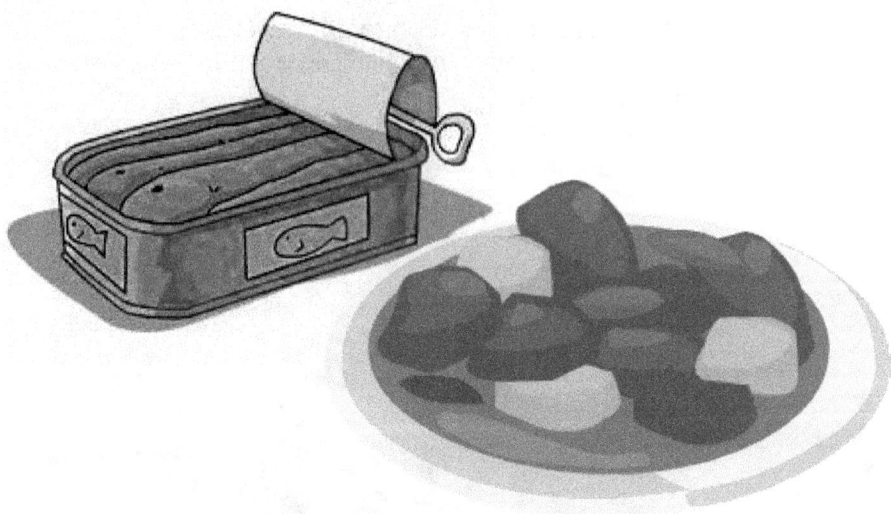

Chili Chicken Sof-Chos (Soft Nachos)

Ingredients:

    1 corn tortilla, shredded
    1 package of chili (cooked or dry; if dry, cook according to instructions below)
    ¼ bag of refried beans
    1 pouch of chicken (shredded or chunked)
    1 squeeze cheese, single serving
    Water
    1 small pot and lid, 1 bowl, 1 spoon (2 pots if cooking dry chili)

Instructions:

1. In the pot, put an equal amount of water as the beans. Bring to a boil and add the beans. Simmer for 5 minutes covered, then let stand for 5 minutes, or according to package directions if other than instant beans are used.
2. If cooking dry chili, put it in the second pot, cover with water, and cook for 20 minutes or according to directions.
3. Rip the tortilla into small pieces and put them into the third bowl.
4. When the beans are done, pour them directly over your tortilla.
5. Open the pouch of chicken. Drain any water and dump the chicken on top of the beans.
6. Open the chili and pour it on top of the chicken.
7. Squirt the cheese over the chili. Dig deep to get a little of everything in each bite.

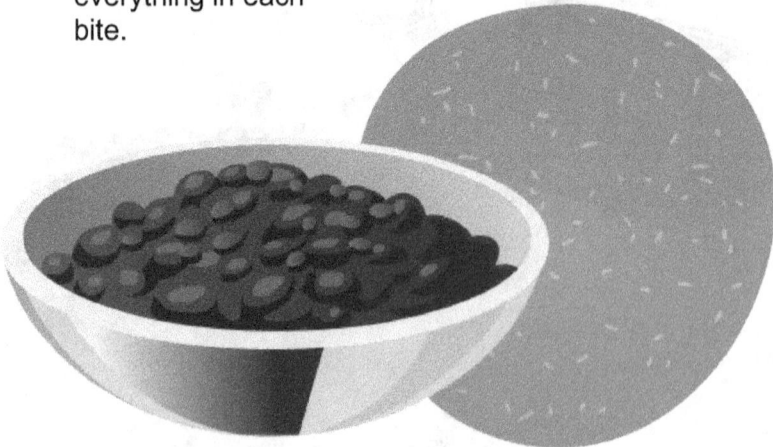

Cheesy Chicken Sof-Chos

Ingredients:
>1 corn tortilla
>1 pouch of chicken (shredded or chunked)
>¼ bag of refried beans
>1 squeeze cheese, single serving
>1 block of cheese, cheddar or mozzarella
>Unlimited jalapenos
>Salsa
>1 small pot and lid, 1 bowl, 1 spoon

Instructions:
1. In the pot, put an equal amount of water as the beans. Bring to a boil and add the beans. Simmer for 5 minutes covered, then let stand for 5 minutes, or according to package directions if other than instant beans are used.
2. In the bowl, take your tortilla and rip it up into small pieces.
3. Cut up the cheese block into small chunks while the beans are cooking.
4. When the beans are done cooking, pour them over the tortilla pieces.
5. Open the chicken pouch, draining the water and dumping the chicken over the beans.
6. Squirt the cheese over the chicken.
7. Put the cheese chunks over the squeezed cheese.
8. Place jalapenos on top, and finally put the salsa over the jalapenos. Spicy!

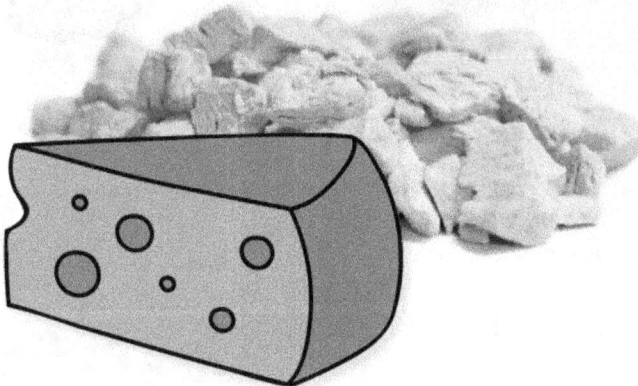

BOB Sof-Chos

Ingredients:
- 1 corn tortilla
- 1 pouch of ready-to-eat chili
- 1 squeeze cheese, single serving
- 1 bowl, 1 spoon

Instructions:
1. Rip the tortilla into small pieces and put them into the first bowl.
2. Open the chili and pour it over the tortilla.
3. Squirt cheese over the chili. This is surprisingly delicious!

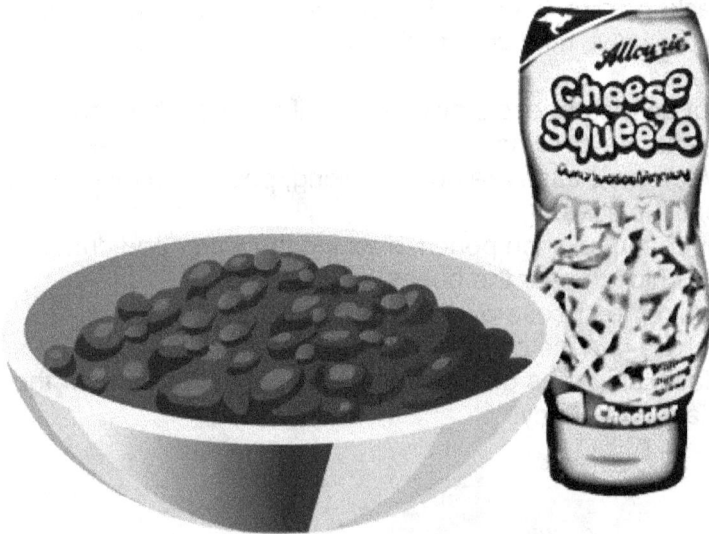

BOB Spicy Sof-Chos

Ingredients:
>1 corn tortilla
>Unlimited jalapenos
>¼ bag of refried beans
>1 squeeze cheese, single serving
>1 small pot and lid, 1 bowl, 1 spoon

Instructions:
1. In the pot, put an equal amount of water as the beans. Bring to a boil and add the beans. Simmer for 5 minutes covered then let stand for 5 minutes, or according to package directions if other than instant beans are used.
2. In the bowl, take the tortilla and rip it up into small pieces into the bowl.
3. When the beans are done, pour them over the tortilla pieces.
4. Squirt cheese over the beans, spreading evenly with a spoon.
5. Add jalapenos on top of the cheese. Don't forget to thank the chef!

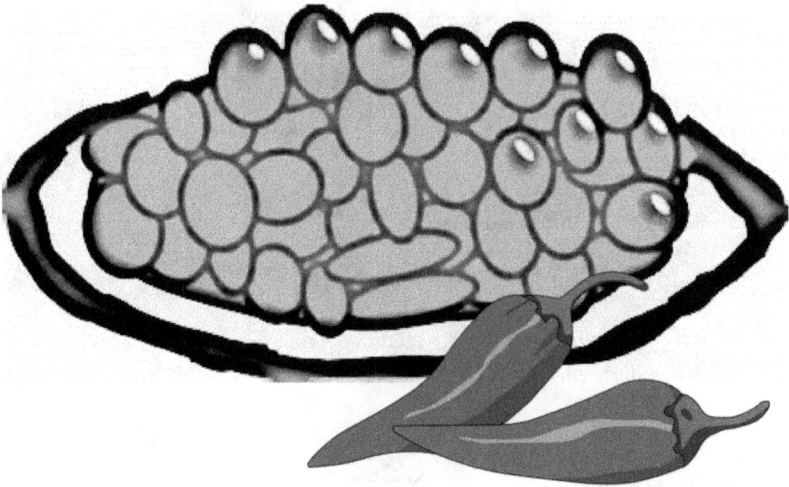

Chubby Sof-Chos

Ingredients:
> 1 corn tortilla
> 1 Lil' Chub, or any spicy meat stick
> ¼ bag of refried beans
> 1 squeeze cheese, single serving
> 1 small pot and lid, 1 bowl, 1 spoon

Instructions:
1. In the pot, put an equal amount of water as the beans. Bring to a boil and add the beans. Simmer for 5 minutes covered, then let stand for 5 minutes, or according to package directions if other than instant beans are used.
2. Rip the tortilla into small pieces and put it into the bowl.
3. When the beans are done cooking, pour them on top of the tortilla pieces.
4. Squeeze the cheese over the beans and spread it evenly with a spoon.
5. Cut up the Lil' Chub and put chunks over the cheese. Chow down!

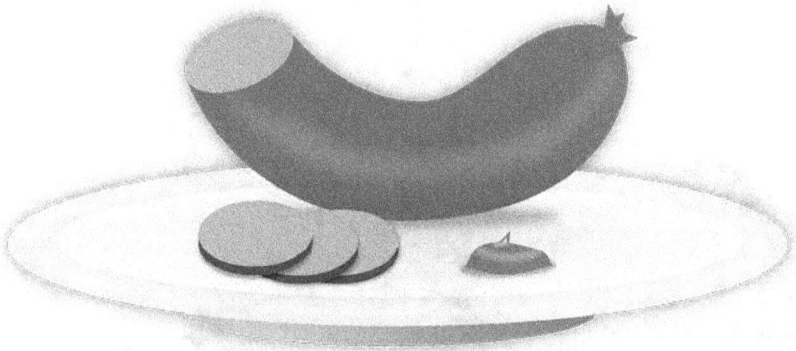

Seafood Poppers Bowl

Ingredients:
> ¼ bag of instant refried beans
> ¼ bag of instant brown rice
> 1 pouch of any fish (tuna, mackerel, sardines, etc.)
> ½ tsp. of garlic powder
> Unlimited jalapenos
> 1 spicy cheese squeeze, single serving
> 1 small pot and lid, 1 bowl, 1 spoon

Instructions:
1. In the pot, put equal amounts of water as the rice and beans. Bring to a boil and add the rice and beans. Simmer for 5 minutes covered, then let stand for 5 minutes, or according to package directions if other than instant rice and beans are used.
2. In the bowl, open the fish, drain the water, and dump the fish into the bowl.
3. Add jalapenos to the fish and stir.
4. When the beans and rice mix is done cooking, take off the lid.
5. Squirt the cheese over the beans.
6. Take your fish and jalapeno bowl and scoop onto the cheese. You'll love it!

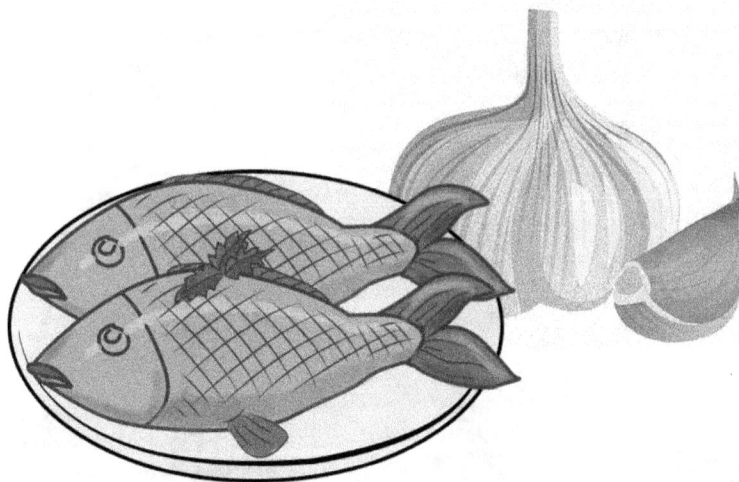

Chickety China Chinese Chicken

Ingredients:
>¼ bag of instant brown rice
>1 spoon of hot sauce or chili garlic sauce
>1 large spoonful of chunky peanut butter
>1 pouch of chicken (shredded or chunked)
>Water
>1 small pot and lid, 1 bowl, 1 cup, 1 spoon

Instructions:
1. Fill a small pot with the same amount of water as the rice being cooked. Heat the water to a boil.
2. Mix the rice and chili garlic sauce in the water and reduce the heat to a simmer for 5 minutes with the lid on the pot. Remove from heat and let stand for 5 minutes until all the water is soaked up by the rice, or cook according to the directions on the package.
3. While the rice is cooking, put peanut butter in the cup. Using hot water, put a very thin layer of water on the peanut butter (about 2 T of water).
4. Stir peanut butter until it is fully mixed with water. It should be about as thick as sauce.
5. When the rice is fully cooked, remove the lid and pour in the peanut sauce. Stir until the sauce is fully blended into the rice.
6. Once combined, open the chicken and drain off any excess water. Dump the meat into the rice. Put a dash of hot sauce over the chicken and rice and stir. Put this all in the bowl. Fire!

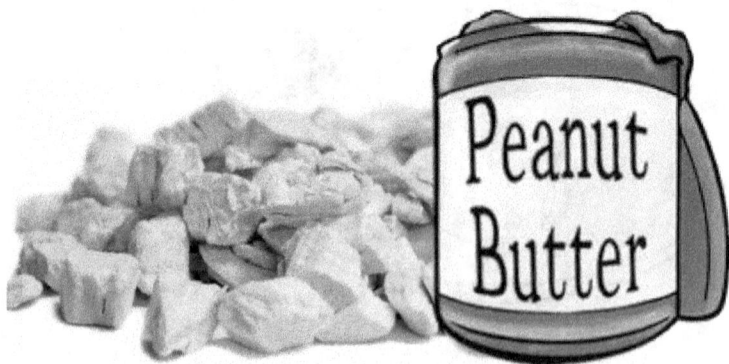

BOB – OG

Ingredients:
> ¼ bag of instant brown rice
> ¼ bag of refried beans
> 1 squeeze cheese, single serving
> Water
> 1 pot and lid, 1 bowl, 1 spoon

Instructions:
1. In the pot, put equal amounts of water as the rice and beans. Bring to a boil and add the rice and beans. Simmer for 5 minutes covered, then let stand for 5 minutes, or according to package directions if other than instant rice and beans are used.
2. Once the beans and rice are fully cooked, squirt the cheese on top, spreading evenly with a spoon.
3. Eat slowly to enjoy fully!

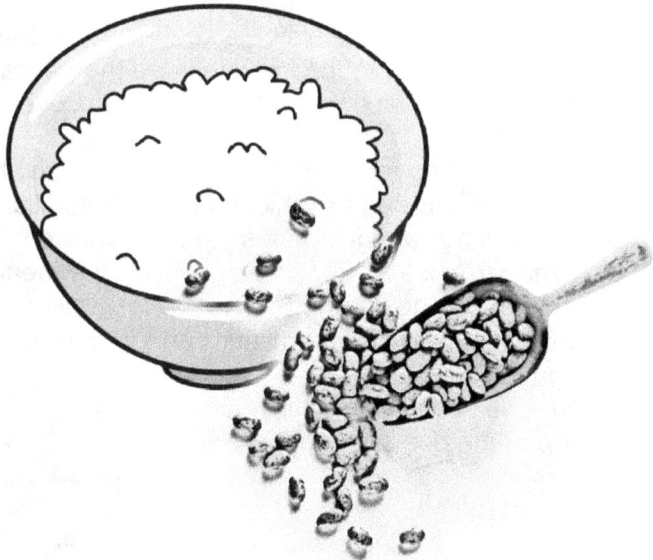

Crazy Rich Peanut Bowl

Ingredients:
>2 corn tortillas
>¼ bag of instant brown rice
>1 pouch of chicken
>1 summer sausage, or large meat stick
>1 pack of unsalted peanuts, 3 oz.
>½ orange Crystal Light
>Peanut trail mix
>Unlimited jalapeno, Hot sauce to taste
>1 squeeze cheese, single serving
>Water
>1 small pot and 2 lids, 1 bowl, 1 spoon

Instructions:
1. Fill a small pot with the same amount of water as the rice being cooked. Heat the water to a boil.
2. Mix the rice in the water along with the orange Crystal Light, reducing the heat to a simmer for 5 minutes with the lid on the pot. Remove from heat and let stand for 5 minutes until all the water is soaked up by the rice, or cook according to the directions on the package.
3. In the bowl, place the tortilla down and cover with a lid. Set aside.
4. While waiting for the rice, open the chicken and drain the liquid off. Spread the chicken over the tortilla.
5. Put trail mix and jalapenos over the chicken.
6. When the rice is fully cooked, cut up the meat, putting it in the rice and stirring.
7. Put the rice and meat mixture on top of the trail mix and jalapenos.
8. Put the second tortilla on top of the rice and meat mixture.
9. Squirt the cheese over the tortilla, spreading evenly with a spoon.
10. Put the unsalted peanuts on top of the cheese. Drizzle hot sauce over the peanuts. You know what's next!

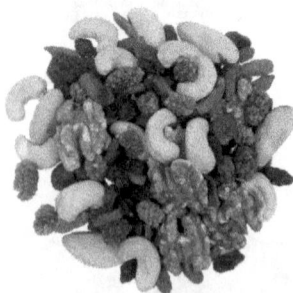

Sour Mack

Ingredients:

      1 pouch mackerel, any brand
      1 pack sweetener (Sweet 'n Low, Equal, Splenda, etc.)
      2 spoonfuls of pickle juice
      Unlimited jalapenos
      1 bag of pork rinds, crushed
      1 bowl, 1 cup, 1 spoon

Instructions:

1. In the cup, add pickle juice, sweetener, and jalapenos. Mix and stir together.
2. Open the mackerel, drain the juice, and dump it into the bowl.
3. Pour the mixture from the cup into the mackerel and combine.
4. Dump the pork rinds into the bowl. That's good eating!

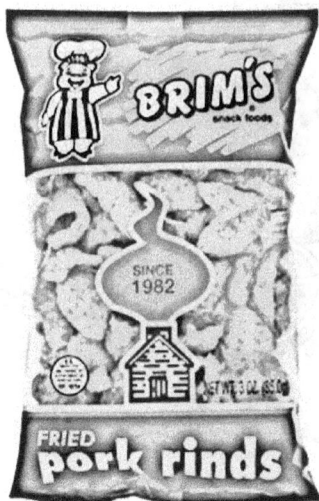

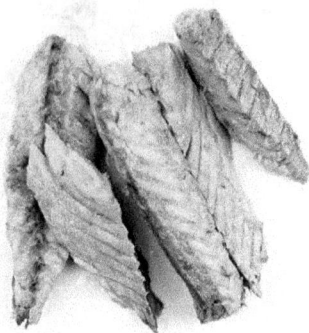

Lemon Fish Lips

Ingredients:
 1 pouch mackerel
 ½ lemon Crystal Light
 ½ spoonful of garlic powder
 ½ spoonful of onion powder
 1 bowl, 1 spoon

Instructions:
 1. Put everything into one bowl.
 2. Mix thoroughly and enjoy!

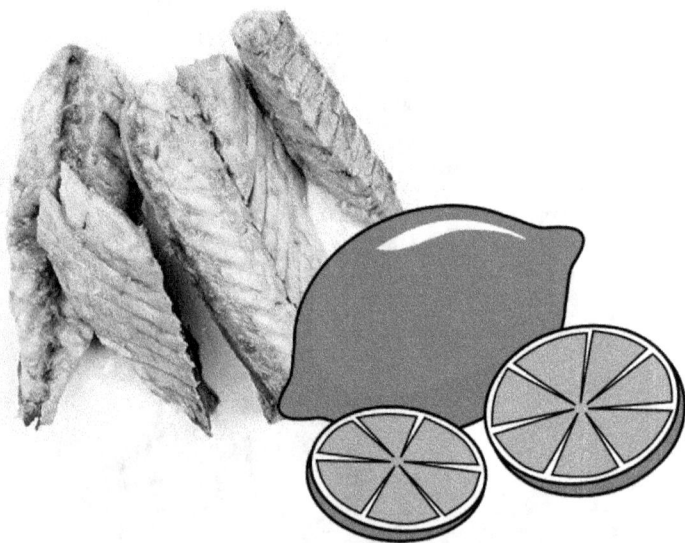

Screamin' Vegan

Ingredients:
- ¼ bag of instant brown rice
- ¼ bag of refried beans
- Hot salsa
- Unlimited jalapeno
- Water
- 1 small pot and lid, 1 bowl, 1 spoon

Instructions:
1. In the pot, put equal amounts of water as the rice and beans. Bring to a boil and add the rice and beans. Simmer for 5 minutes covered, then let stand for 5 minutes, or according to package directions if other than instant rice and beans are used.
2. Once fully cooked, take off the lid and pour hot salsa on top.
3. Add jalapenos on top of the salsa and spread evenly. Hot, hot, hot!

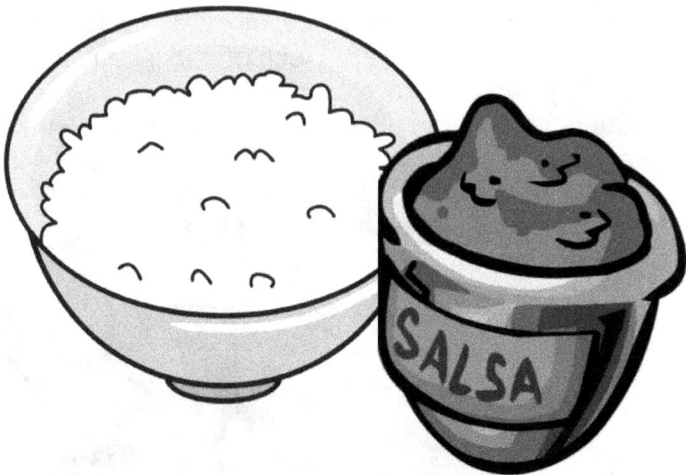

3-Rex

Ingredients:
- ¼ bag of instant brown rice
- ½ spoonful of garlic powder
- 1 meat stick of any kind
- 1 pouch of chicken
- 1 pouch of mackerel
- 1 squeeze cheese, single serving
- 1 pickle, diced
- Water
- 1 small pot and lid, 1 bowl, 1 spoon

Instructions:
1. Fill a small pot with the same amount of water as the rice being cooked. Heat the water to a boil.
2. Mix the rice in the water and reduce the heat to a simmer for 5 minutes with the lid on the pot. Remove from heat and let stand for 5 minutes until all the water is soaked up by the rice, or cook according to the directions on the package.
3. While waiting for the rice, cut up the meat stick into small chunks and cut up the pickle into small chunks. Put them into the bowl. Open the mackerel, drain the juice, and add it to the meat and pickle mixture. Mix together well.
4. When the rice is cooked, take off the lid and add the garlic powder. Mix well.
5. Squirt cheese over the garlic rice. Spread evenly with a spoon.
6. Carefully combine the rice and meat mixture. I like meat on the bottom, rice on the top. Mix and stir if you like! Either way, 3 times the meat equals 3 times delicious!

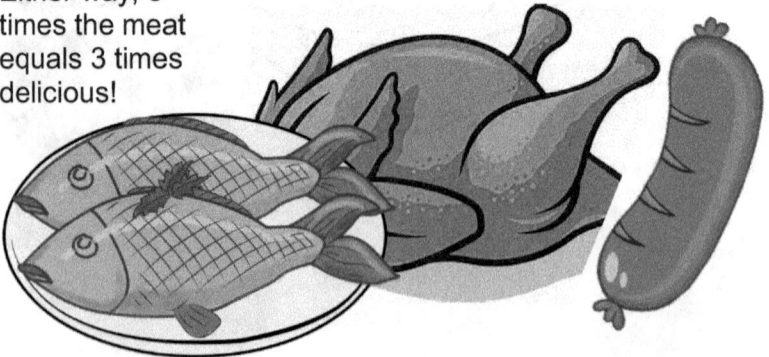

Egg Salad

Ingredients:

> 4 boiled eggs or 1 pack of microwavable egg powder
> 2 mustard singles or 2 tsp. spoonfuls of prepared mustard
> 2 mayonnaise singles or 2 spoonfuls of mayonnaise
> ¼ pickle, diced
> 1 squeeze cheese, single serving
> 2 bowls, 1 spoon

Instructions:

1. Put the eggs in the first bowl and smash them into crumbles. For microwavable eggs, follow the label instructions.
2. In the second bowl, add the mayonnaise, mustard, and pickle.
3. Add smashed eggs to the second bowl.
4. Mix thoroughly until everything is blended well. You're going to love it!

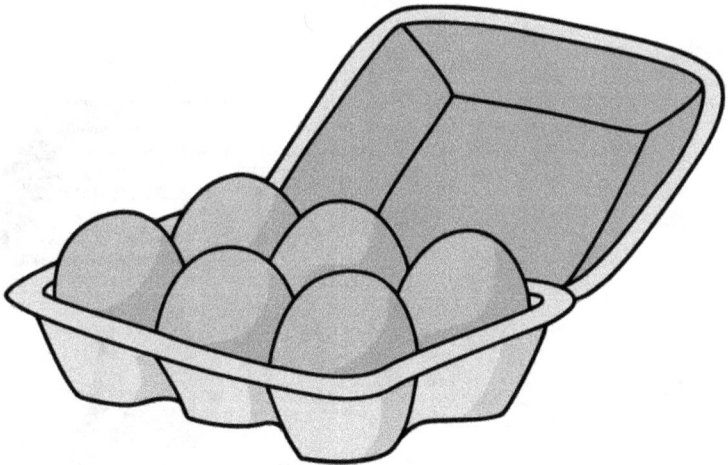

Loaded Jalapeno Bowl

Ingredients
¼ bag of refried beans
1 pack of cream cheese, single serving
1 squeeze cheese, single serving
Unlimited jalapenos
Water
1 small pot and lid, 1 bowl, 1 spoon

Instructions:
1. In the pot, put an equal amount of water as the beans. Bring to a boil and add the beans. Simmer for 5 minutes covered, then let stand for 5 minutes, or according to package directions if other than instant beans are used.
2. In the bowl, put a layer of jalapenos down to act as a crust.
3. When the beans are done cooking, add cream cheese, mixing well.
4. Carefully pour the bean mixture onto the jalapenos.
5. Squirt cheese over the beans, spreading evenly with a spoon. Do not share!

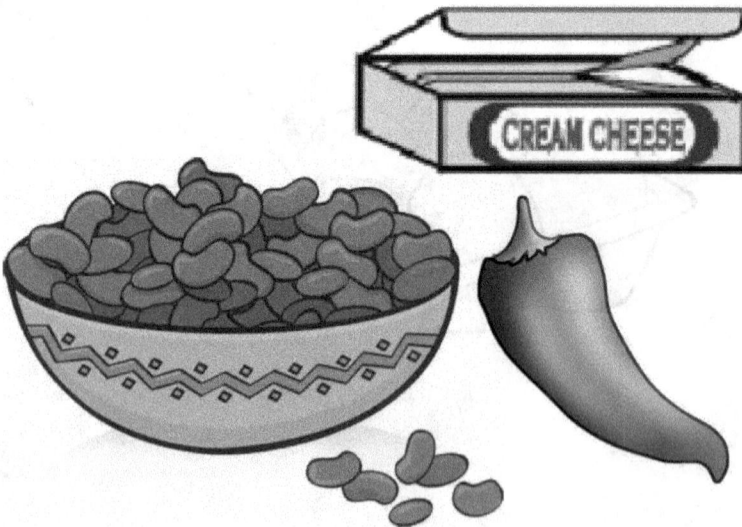

Far East Tuna

Ingredients:

¼ bag of instant brown rice
1 pouch of tuna, any brand
¼ pickle, diced
1 pack of mustard, single serving or 1 spoonful of mustard
1 spicy squeeze cheese, single serving
2 spoonfuls of soy sauce
Water
1 small pot and lid, 1 bowl, 1 spoon

Instructions:

1. Fill a small pot with the same amount of water as the rice being cooked. Heat the water to a boil.
2. Mix the rice in the water and reduce the heat to a simmer for 5 minutes with the lid on the pot. Remove from heat and let stand for 5 minutes until all the water is soaked up by the rice, or cook according to the directions on the package.
3. In the bowl, dump in the tuna, mustard, and diced pickle, and mix together.
4. Once rice is cooked, take off the lid and add soy sauce. Mix well.
5. Once combined, add the tuna mixture to the rice. Stir together. Squirt cheese over the tuna-rice mixture. Spread the cheese evenly on top with a spoon. Pat yourself on the back!

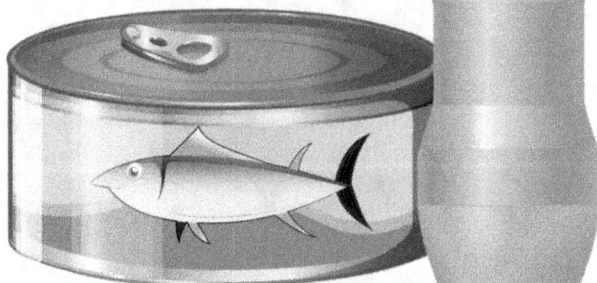

Meat Shell Tacos

Ingredients:
2 meat sticks
¼ block of mozzarella or cheddar cheese
4 jalapeno wheels, diced (optional)
1 bowl, 1 spoon, 1 ruler

Instructions:
1. Carefully slice the meat stick down the middle, making sure not to cut all the way through.
2. Cut the cheese into slim, long pieces and place them into the meat stick.
3. Scatter diced jalapeno onto the cheese. Everyone will be doing it soon!

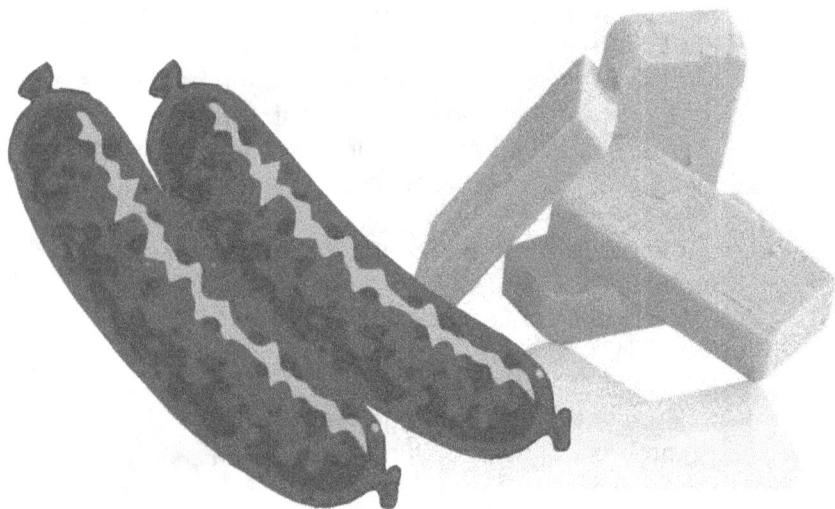

Tuna Crunch

Ingredients:
       1 pouch tuna, drained
       1 bag nuts, peanuts, cashews, sunflower seeds, etc.
       1 handful of raisins
       1 bowl, 1 spoon

Instructions:
1. Put all the ingredients in the bowl and stir. So good!

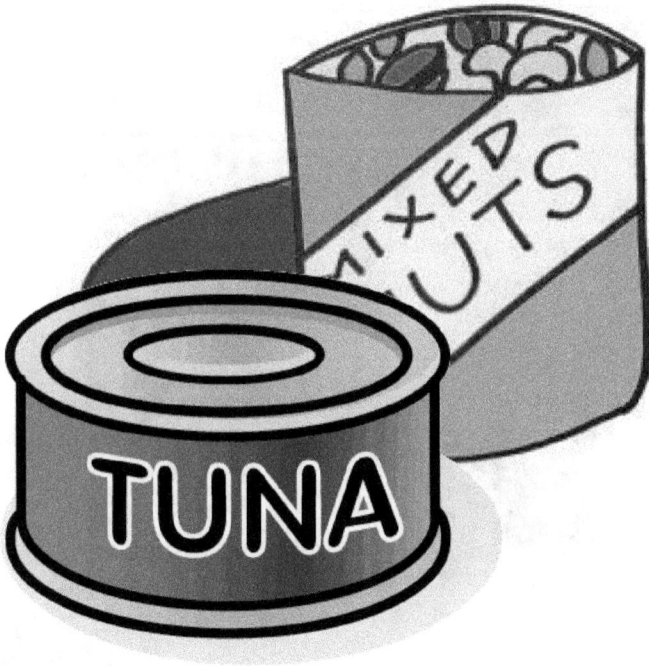

Fruit & Chicken Salad

Ingredients:
>1 pouch of chicken, shredded or chunk
>1 packet mayonnaise, single serving
>½ apple, peeled and cut up
>1 handful of raisins
>1 spoon of prepared mustard
>Pepper to taste
>1 bowl, 1 spoon

Instructions:
1. Put everything in a bowl and stir together until well blended. Enjoy!

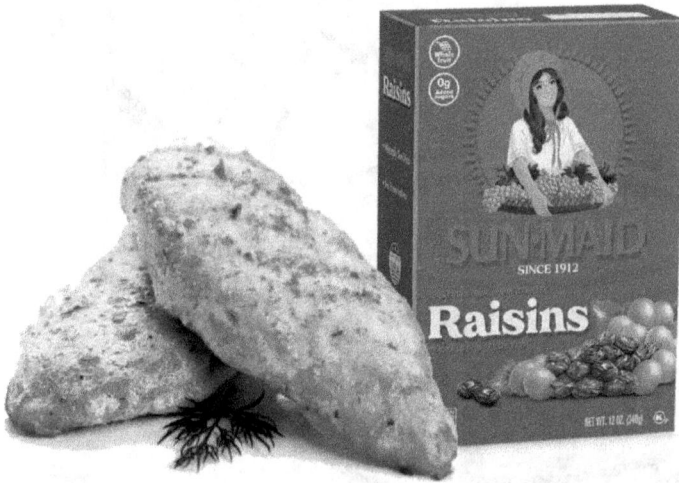

Health Bowl

Ingredients:
    ¼ bag of instant brown rice
    1 bag trail mix
    3 spoonfuls of raisins
    ¼ tsp. of cinnamon
    Water
    1 small pot and lid, 1 bowl, 1 spoon

Instructions:
1. Fill a small pot with the same amount of water as the rice being cooked. Heat the water to a boil.
2. Mix the rice in the water and reduce the heat to a simmer for 5 minutes with the lid on the pot. Remove from heat and let stand for 5 minutes until all the water is soaked up by the rice, or cook according to the directions on the package.
3. Once the rice is cooked, open the trail mix and pour it into the rice. Mix together.
4. Once combined, put in the bowl and top with raisins evenly.
5. Garnish with cinnamon. Top of the morning!

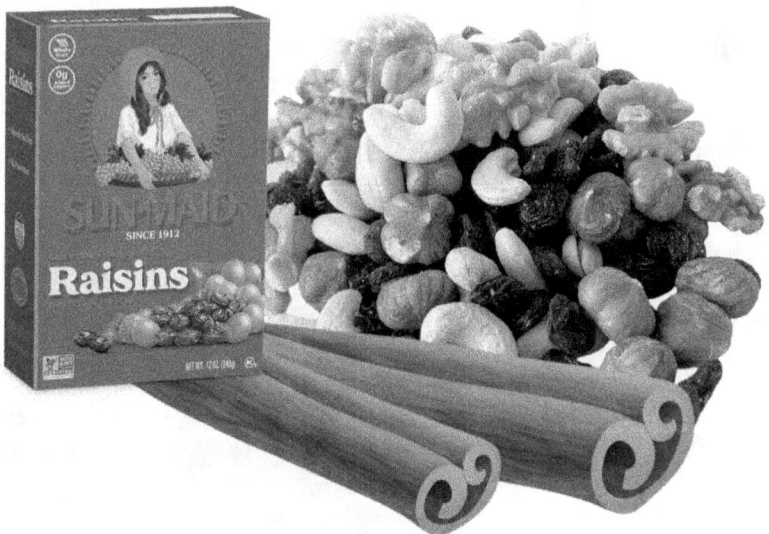

CHAPTER TWO

Healthy Drinks

Funny Juice

Ingredients:
>Hot water
>2 spoonfuls of Colombian coffee
>1 fruit punch Crystal Light (or any like-brand), single serving
>1 cup

Instructions:
1. In the cup, add coffee and Crystal Light.
2. Add hot water until halfway full.
3. Add ice for the other half; if no ice is available, use cold water until the cup is full. Drink up!

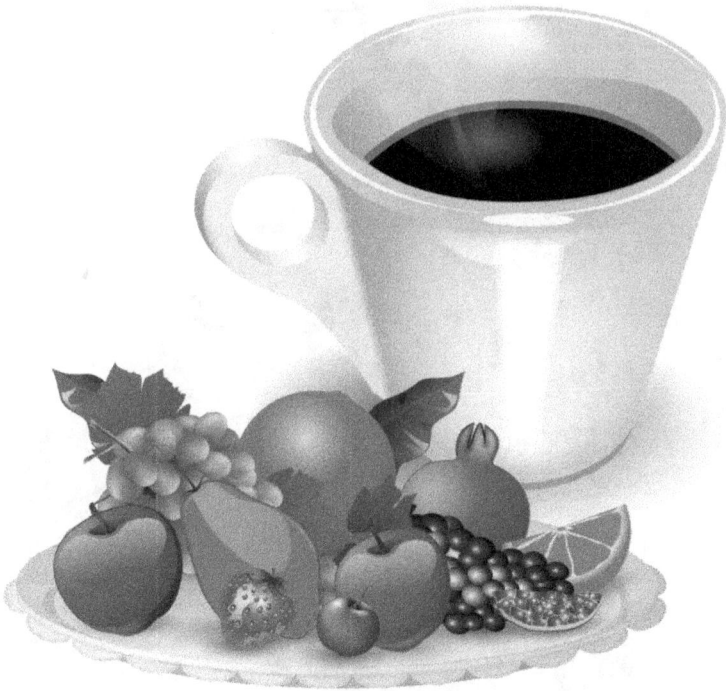

Dragon Tea

Ingredients:
>Hot water
>2 tea bags of black tea
>1 orange Crystal Light (or any brand), single serving
>2 cups

Instructions:
1. In the first cup, brew the tea using hot water. Let the tea brew for 15 minutes or to your liking.
2. In the second cup, add orange Crystal Light. Add just a dash of hot water and stir. (Use no more than 2 spoonfuls of water to mix with the Crystal Light.)
3. Once the tea is brewed, pour the orange mixture into the tea. Enjoy

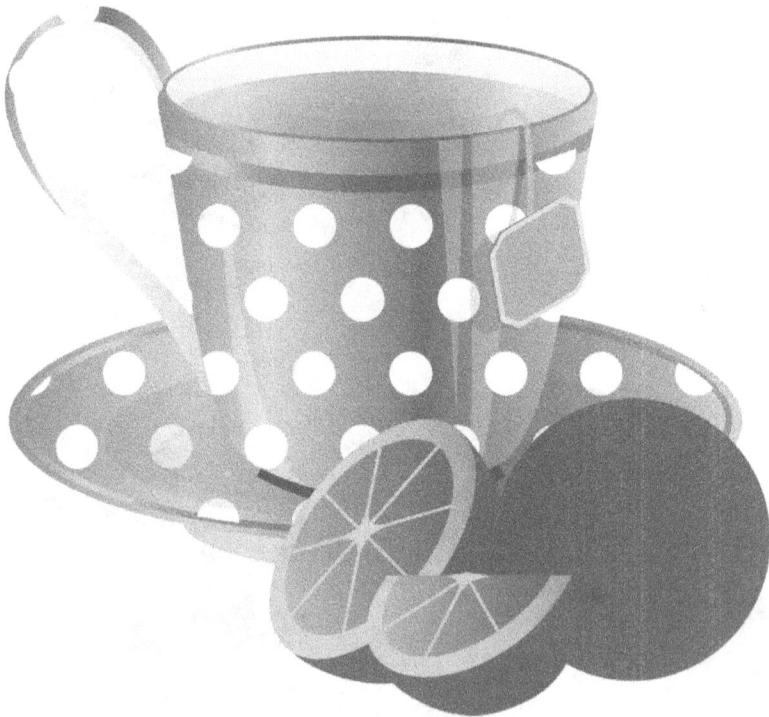

Hybrid Caddy

Ingredients:
> Hot water
> 2 tea bags of black tea
> 2 spoonfuls of Colombian coffee
> 1 sugar-free cocoa packet
> 2 cups

Instructions:
1. First, fill halfway with hot water and insert tea bags. Let the tea brew for 15 minutes, or to your liking.
2. In the second cup, add coffee and cocoa, then add hot water until the cup is ⅓ full.
3. When the tea is done brewing, pour in the coffee-cocoa mixture.
4. Stir and sip!

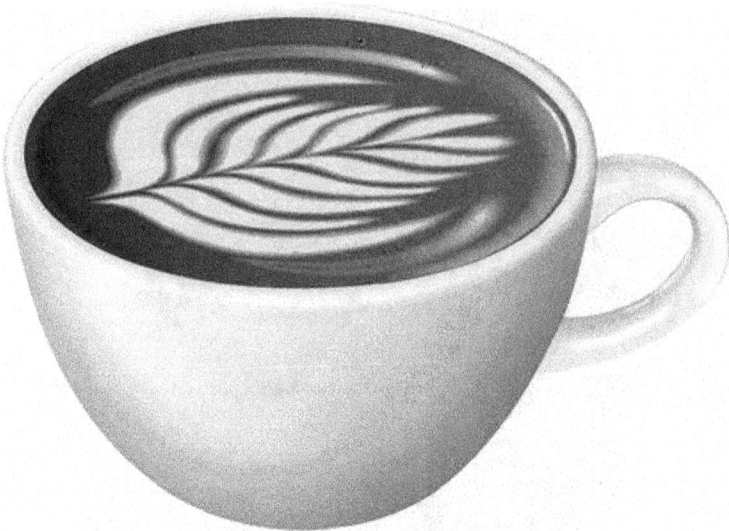

Mocha Cappuccino

Ingredients:
- Hot water
- 2 spoonfuls of Colombian coffee
- 3 spoonfuls of low-fat powdered milk
- 1 sugar-free cocoa packet
- 1 sweetener
- 1 cup

Instructions:
1. In the cup, add all the ingredients at once.
2. Add hot water until cup is full. (The less water you add, the stronger the drink will be!) Cappuccino delicio!

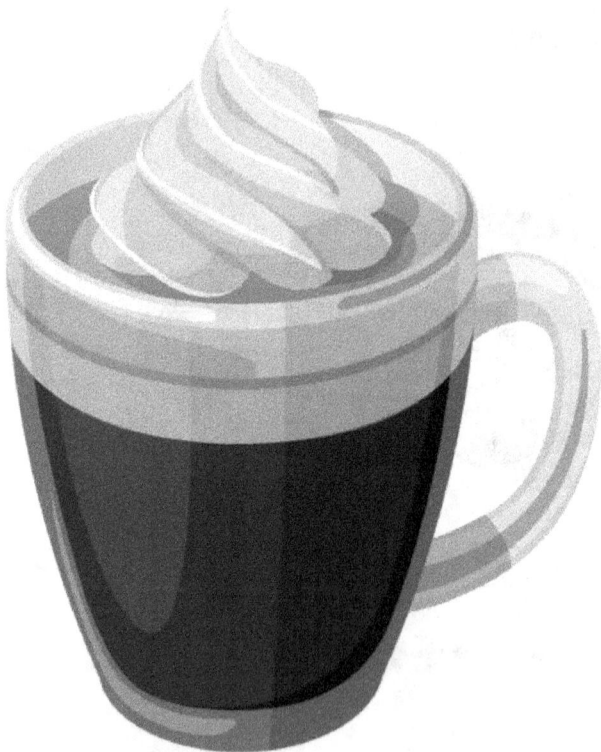

Moo-Tea

Ingredients:
Hot water
2 black tea bags
1 orange Crystal Light, or any comparable brand
2 spoonfuls of low-fat powdered milk
2 cups

Instructions:
1. In one cup, brew tea using hot water. Let it brew for 15 minutes.
2. In another cup, add powdered milk and follow directions to reconstitute.
3. Once the tea is brewed, remove the tea bag, pour in Crystal Light powder and stir.
4. Now, combine your milk and orange tea. Very soothing!

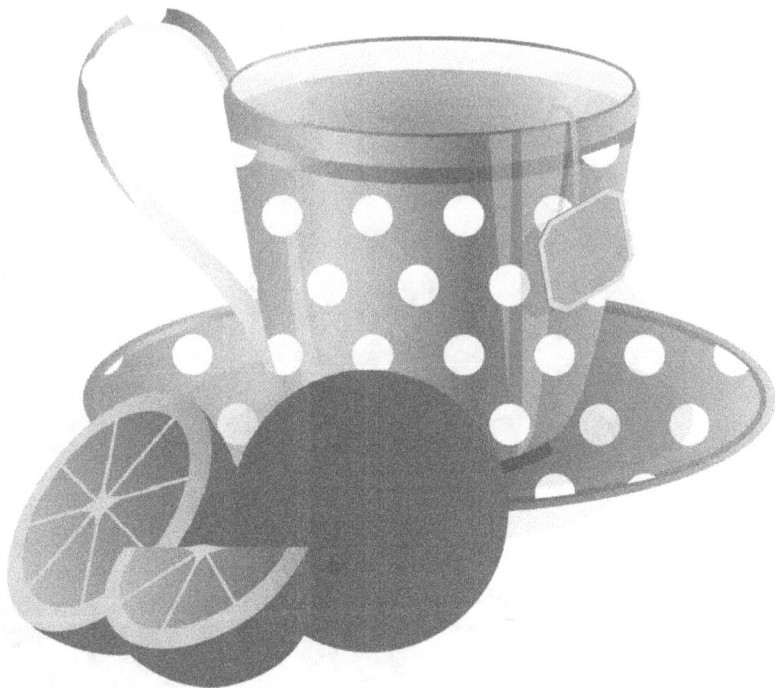

Chai-T

Ingredients:
Hot water
1 bag of black tea
2 spoonfuls of powdered milk
¼ tsp. of cinnamon
2 cups

Instructions:
1. In the first cup, fill halfway with hot water. Add a tea bag and let it brew for 5-10 minutes.
2. While waiting for the tea to brew, add milk and cinnamon to the second cup, mixing while dry. Then add water until the cup is almost half full.
3. When the tea is done brewing to your liking, pour the milk and cinnamon mixture into it. Enjoy!

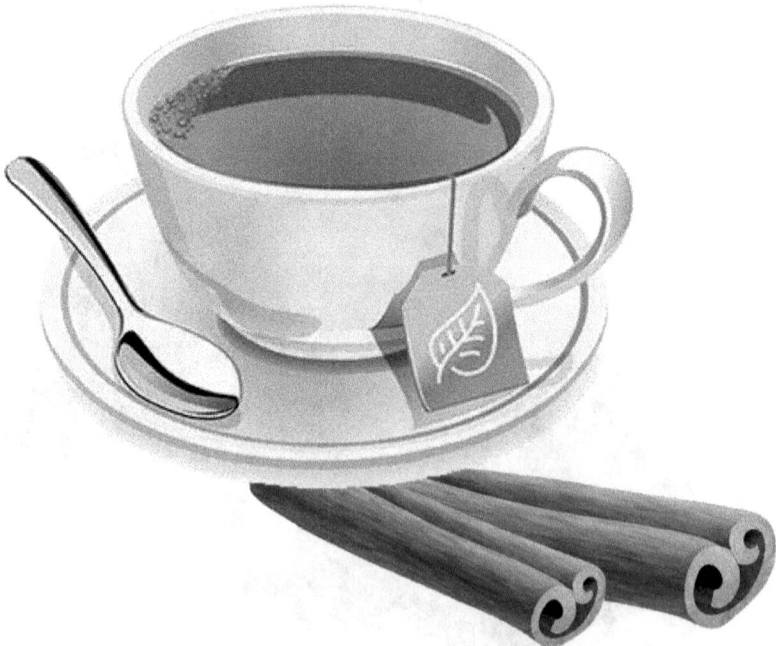

Lemon Iced Tea

Ingredients:
>Hot water
>2 tea bags, black
>1 lemon Crystal Light, or comparable brand
>Ice
>2 cups

Instructions:
1. Fill the first cup completely full of hot water. Insert both tea bags and let it brew for 10 minutes.
2. Fill the second cup with ice.
3. Add Crystal Light however you wish, either over the ice or into the brewing tea.
4. When the tea is fully brewed, pour the hot tea over ice and stir. There will be extra tea, so when you finish drinking your first cup, get more ice and pour the rest. A classic drink!

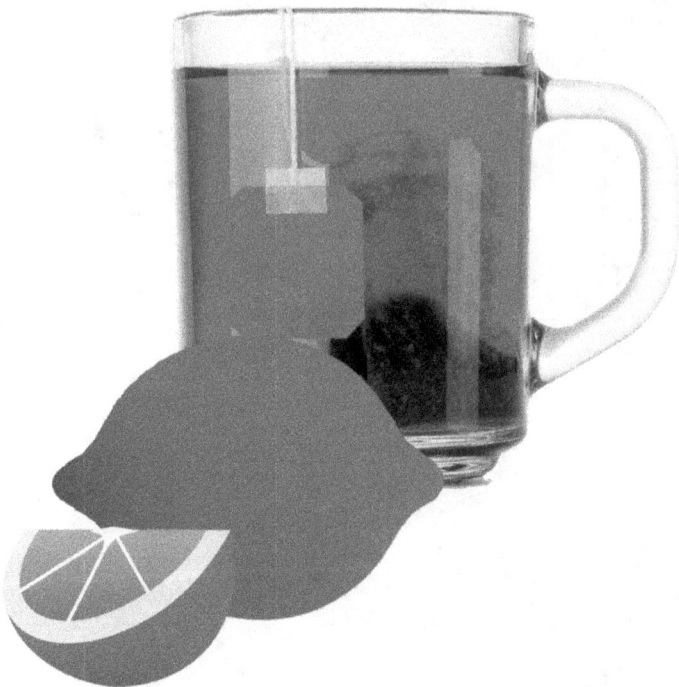

Cinna Milk

Ingredients:
>
> Hot water
> 3 spoonfuls of powdered milk
> ¼ tsp. of cinnamon
> 1 sweetener
> 1 cup

Instructions:
1. Put all the ingredients in the cup.
2. Stir together while dry to combine well.
3. Add hot water and stir. Moo-licious!

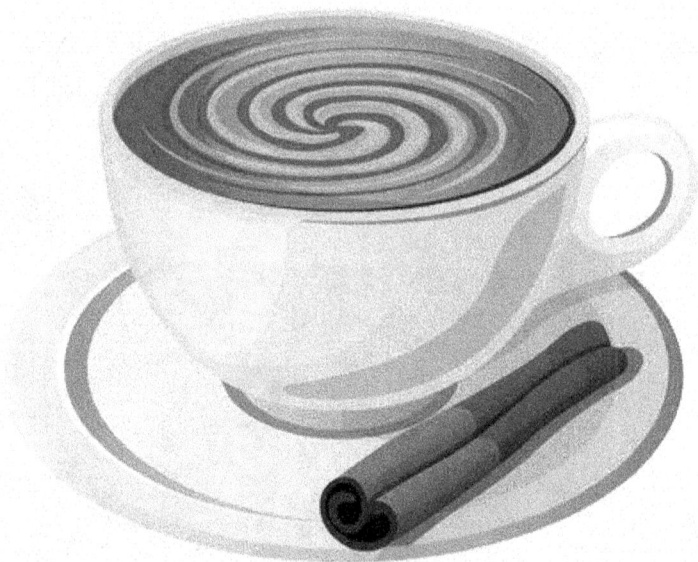

Flavor Fusions

Ingredients:
> Water
> 2 or more Crystal Light (or any brand of different flavors), single serving
> 1 cup

Instructions:
> 1. Combine 2 or more Crystal Light packets in a cup and add water. Stir well to blend.

Here are some of my favorites:

- Raspberry Lemonade & Lemonade
- Iced Tea & Lemonade
- Iced Tea & Raspberry Ice
- Raspberry Ice & Lemonade
- Iced Tea & Orange
- Cherry Pomegranate (Welch's) & Raspberry Lemonade
- Blue Typhoon (Hawaiian Punch) & Green Apple Sour (Jolly Rancher)
- Cherry (Jolly Rancher) & Lemonade
- Fruit Punch & Orange
- Peach Tea & Iced Tea

*Make sure you use sugar-free singles.

Experiment with different flavors and feel the fusion!

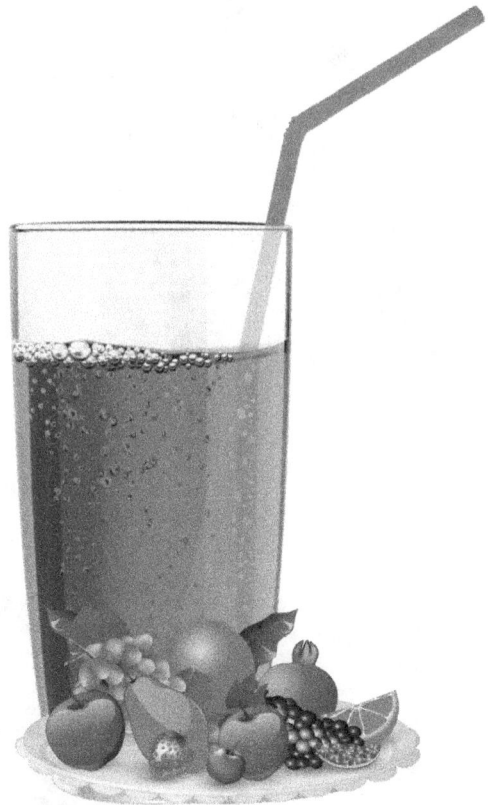

Tiger Milk

Ingredients:
Water
3 spoonfuls of powdered milk
1 orange Crystal Light (any brand)
1 cup

Instructions:
1. Add the ingredients to your cup.
2. Stir while dry to mix evenly.
3. Add water and stir. You might have to dissolve the milk in a small amount of warm water first to get it to dissolve well. Wow!

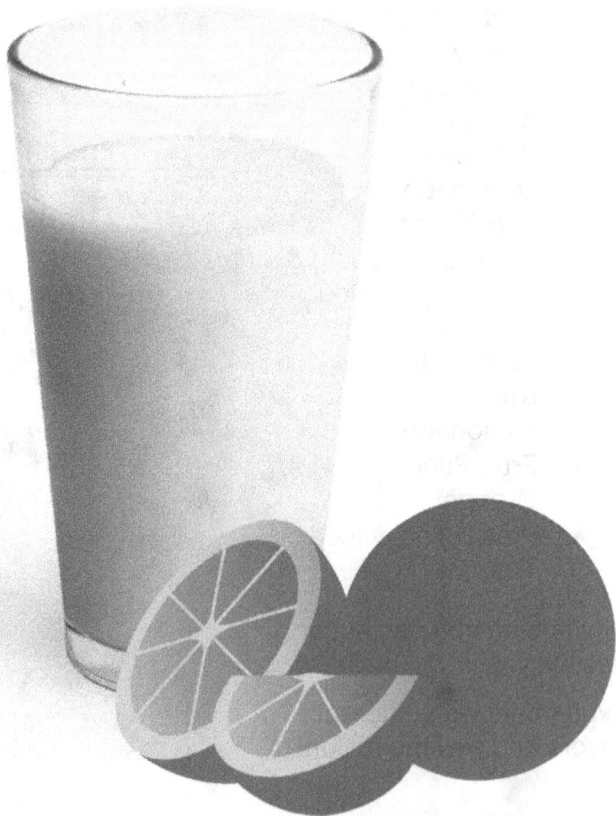

Rush Hour

Ingredients:
   Hot water
   2 tea bags, black
   2 spoonfuls of any instant coffee
   2 cups

Instructions:
   1. Brew the tea in the first cup with 8 oz. (1 cup) of water for 10 minutes.
   2. Make the coffee in the second cup using 2 oz. of water. The coffee will be thick. Add more water if desired.
   3. When the tea is finished, pour it into the coffee cup.

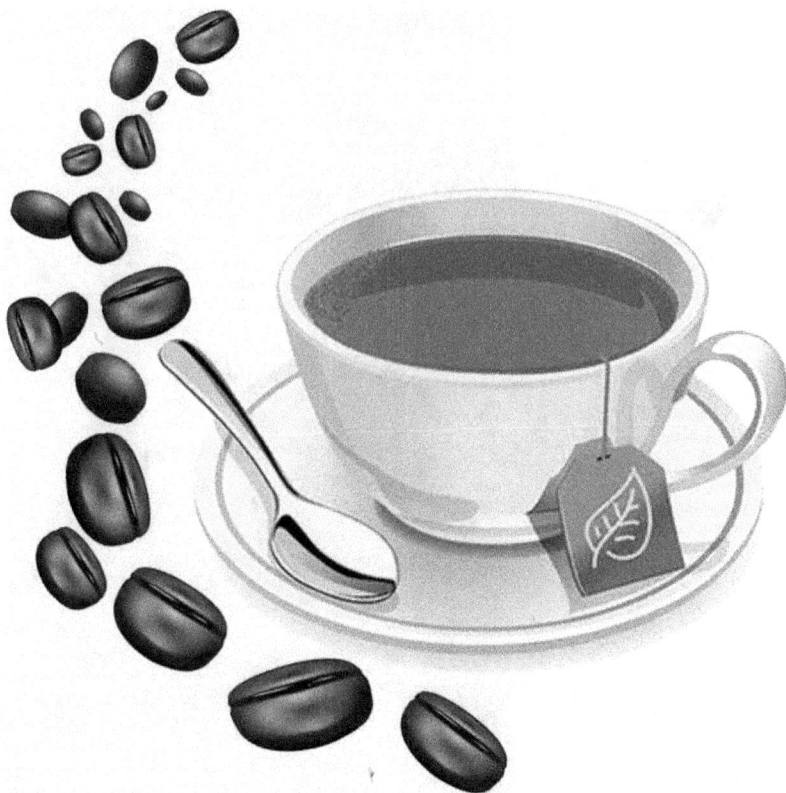

Creamy Cocoa

Ingredients:
Hot water
2 spoonfuls of powdered milk
1 packet or 3 spoonfuls of sugar-free cocoa
1 cup

Instructions:
1. Add all the ingredients to the cup.
2. Stir while dry to produce an even mixture.
3. Add hot water and stir.
4. Let cool for 3-5 minutes. Enjoy!

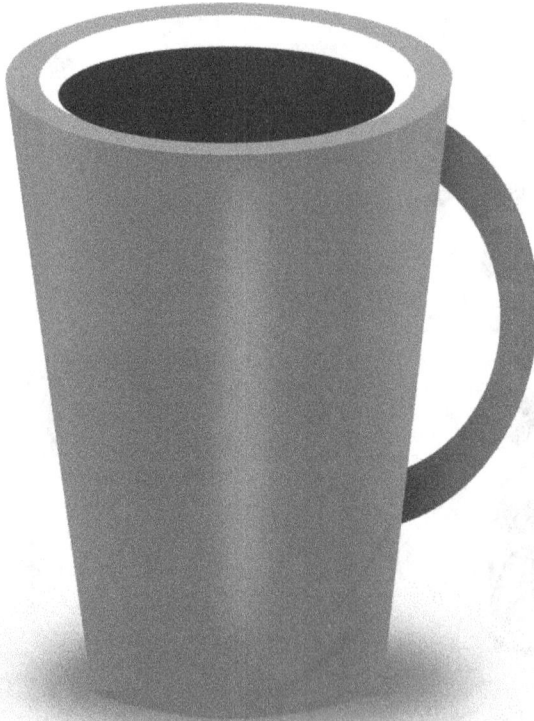

Groovy Smoothies

Ingredients:
Hot water
1 fruit punch Crystal Light, or any brand, single serving
2 spoonfuls of non-dairy creamer powder
1 sweetener
Ice
1 cup

Instructions:
1. Add all the ingredients into the cup, except the ice.
2. Stir the dry ingredients for a more even mixture.
3. Add hot water until the cup is *under* half full.
4. Add ice until the cup is nearly full.
5. Stir the ice in the cup and enjoy.

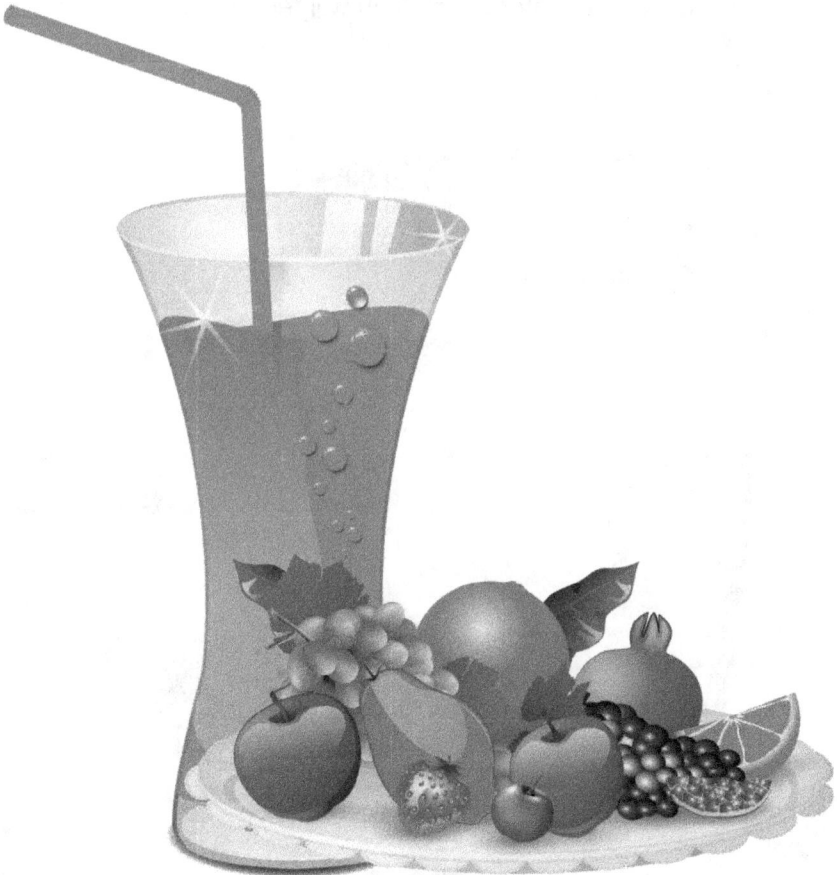

The Flood Gate – For Digestive Movement

Ingredients:
> Water
> Fiber powder
> Crystal Light
> 1 cup

Instructions:
1. Add fiber powder and Crystal Light to the cup (check dosing to see what amount of fiber you need).
2. Mix while dry.
3. Add water and stir.
4. Chug the drink mix down.
5. Refill the cup with water and stir, making sure to get any fiber powder that may stick to the sides.
6. Chug the water down. You will feel better soon!

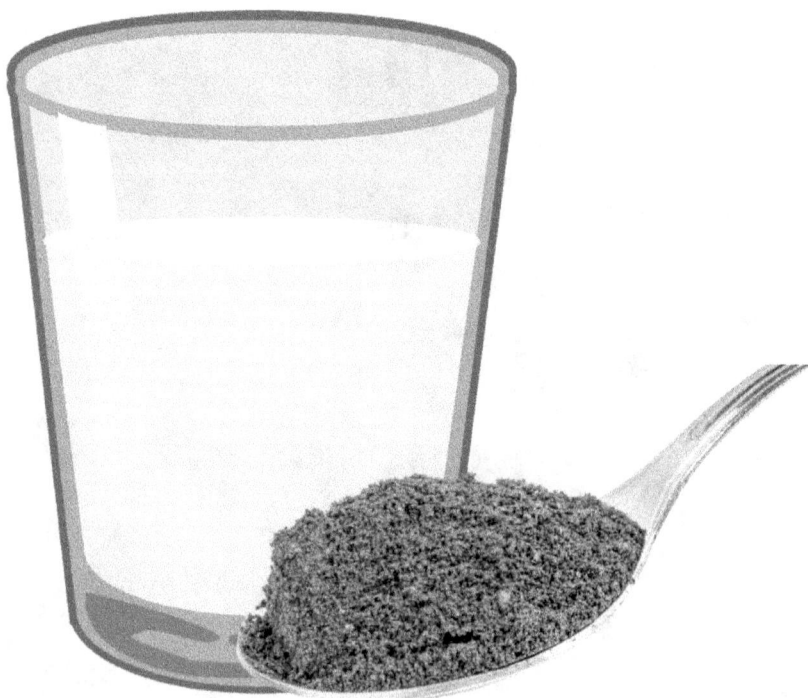

Soothe Aide

Ingredients:
> Hot water
> 2 tea bags, black
> 1 lemon or cherry cough drop
> 1 cup, 1 spoon

Instructions:
1. Crush the cough drop and put it in the cup.
2. Run hot water over the cough drop until it is slightly covered.
3. Use the spoon to stir the cough drop until it melts.
4. Once it is melted, fill the cup with hot water.
5. Insert tea bags and let them brew for 15 minutes. Sip slowly. Get well soon!

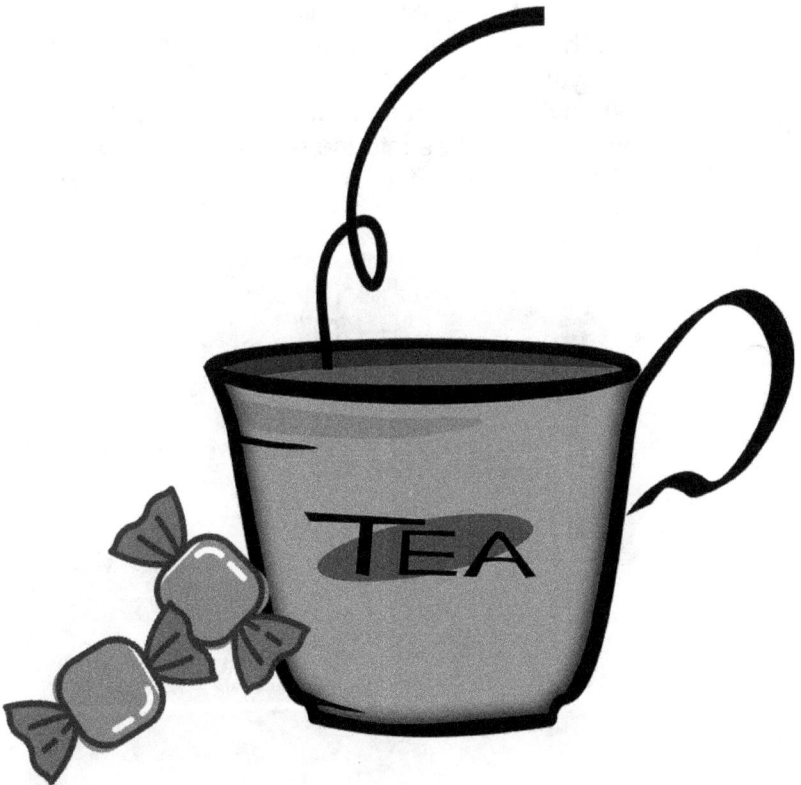

The Smack Down

Ingredients:
Hot water
2 scoops of coffee
2 tea bags, black
2 scoops powdered milk
1 packet or 3 scoops of sugar-free cocoa
½ tsp. of cinnamon
2 large cups

Instructions:
1. In the first cup, add cinnamon and tea bags. Fill the cup halfway with hot water and let it brew for 10 minutes.
2. In the second cup, add the coffee, cocoa, and powdered milk, mixing well.
3. Add half a cup of hot water and stir, making sure everything dissolves.
4. When the tea is done brewing, combine the 2 cups by pouring coffee into the tea or vice versa. Enjoy all of the flavors!

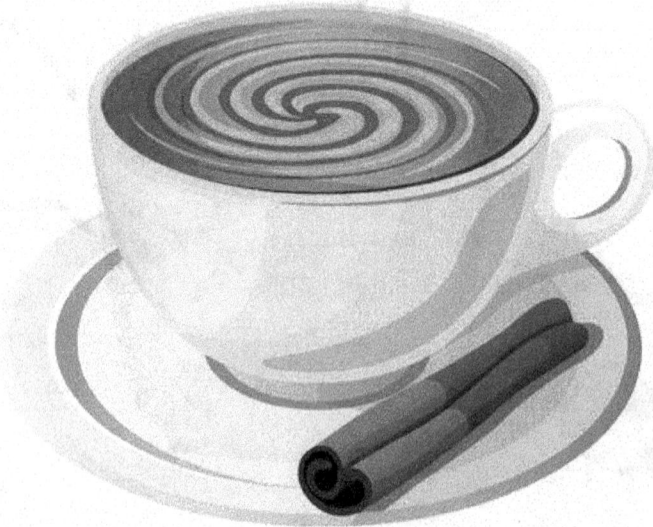

"It's when you run away that you are most likely to stumble."
– Casey Robinson

Thinking that you have lost before the game is over is a loss in itself. Even when the chips are down, keep fighting. Sometimes you might step on the scale after a vigorous week of exercise and eating right, only to find that the scale might be up a pound or two. Don't give up. It could be body weight fluctuation, water weight, or even certain clothes you have on. Don't let that deter you. Don't let anything deter you. There is never a good reason to give up on your goals.

CHAPTER THREE

Healthy Sweet Treats

No Bake Bowl

Ingredients:

Water
⅓ bowl or ½ tumbler of dry instant oatmeal
2 packets or 6 scoops of sugar-free cocoa
1 spoonful of crunchy peanut butter
1 bowl or 1 tumbler cup

Instructions:

1. Mix all ingredients in a bowl using enough water to combine everything, but not enough to make it soupy. Use a little water at a time until it gets absorbed, then add more.
2. Once everything is mixed together, let it stand for 20 minutes covered, but not airtight/pressed fully down. Dig in!

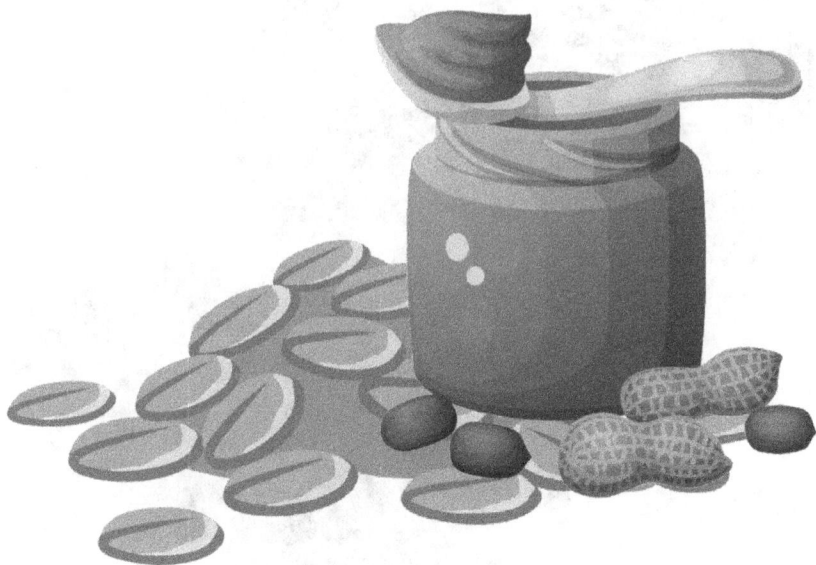

Fruity Oatmeal

Ingredients:
>Hot water
>Any fruit flavored Crystal Light, any brand
>Half a bowl of instant oatmeal
>1 bowl

Instructions:
1. Put the oatmeal in the bowl, and empty the Crystal Light over the oatmeal.
2. Add hot water according to package directions and stir. This is very tasty!

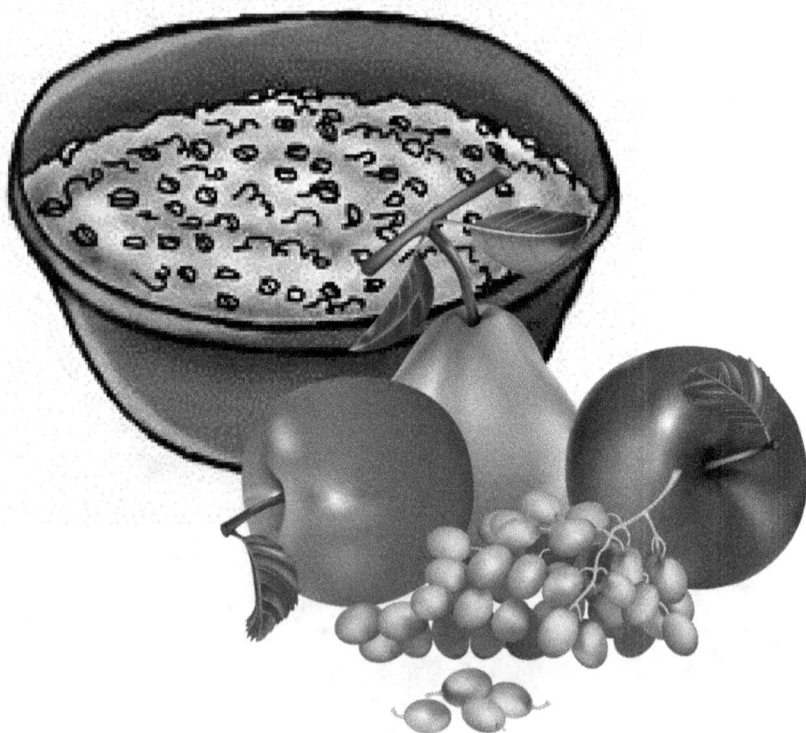

Cinna Rice

Ingredients:
> Hot water
> ¼ bag of instant brown rice
> ¼ tsp. of cinnamon
> Raisins, optional
> 1 small pot and lid. 1 bowl

Instructions:
1. Fill a small pot with the same amount of water as the rice being cooked. Heat the water to a boil.
2. Mix the rice in the water and reduce the heat to a simmer for 5 minutes with the lid on the pot. Remove from heat and let stand for 5 minutes until all the water is soaked up by the rice, or cook according to the directions on the package.
3. When the rice is done cooking, add cinnamon to the rice. If you'd like, add raisins as well and stir. Enjoy!

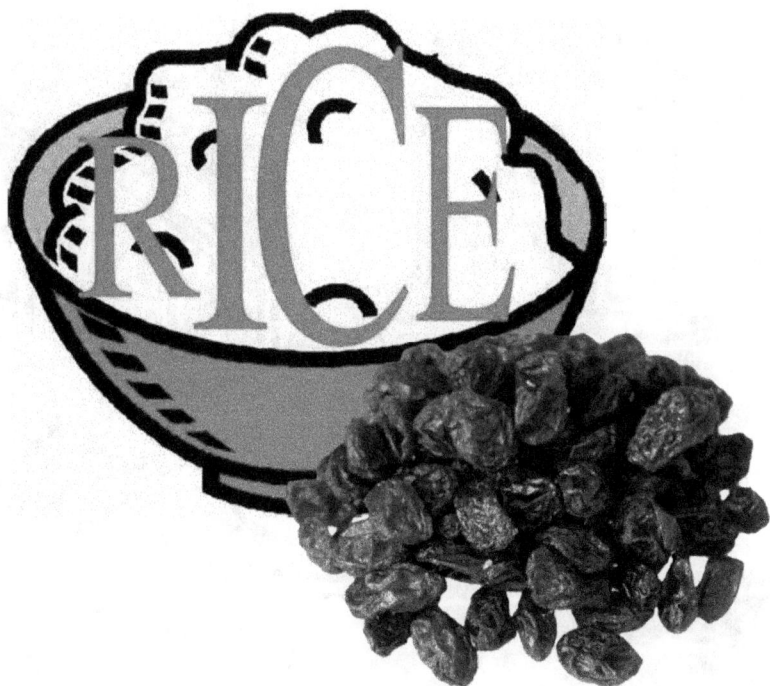

PBR (Peanut Butter Raisin) Oatmeal

Ingredients:
Hot water
Half a bowl of instant oatmeal
2 scoops of peanut butter (crunchy or creamy)
1 handful of raisins
1 small pot, 1 bowl

Instructions:
1. In the pot, add water in the suggested amount given on the package and heat to a boil. Cook according to directions.
2. Pour the oatmeal into the bowl.
3. Spread peanut butter evenly over the top of the oatmeal.
4. Sprinkle the raisins over the peanut butter or decorate with a happy face, star, your initials, etc. This is a great snack.

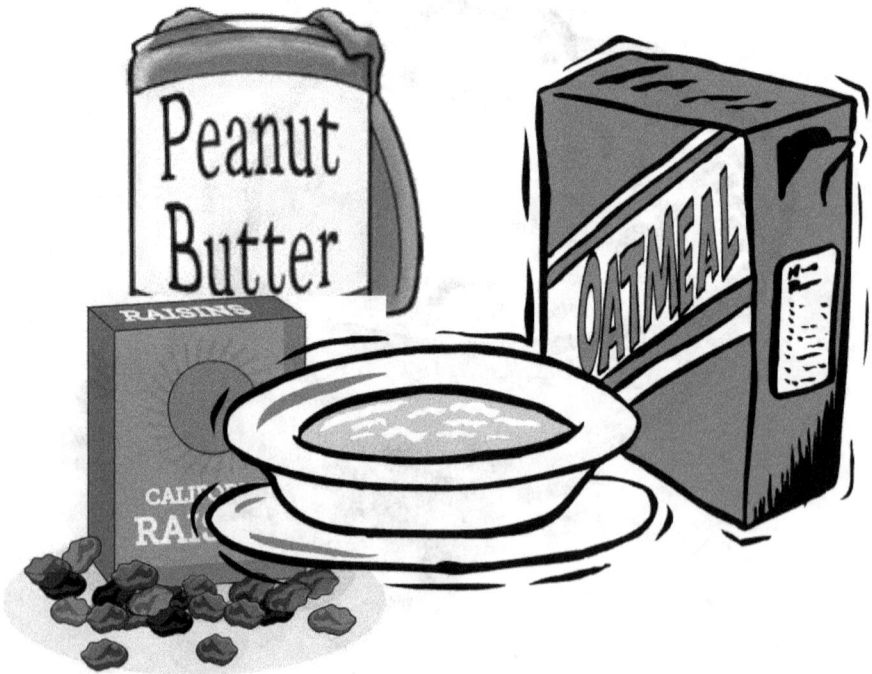

Raisin Sun

Ingredients:
>1 fun size bag of sunflower seeds
>½ cup of raisins
>1 cup or bowl

Instructions:
>1. Place all ingredients in the cup or bowl.
>2. Place a lid on it and shake well using one hand to hold the lid down.
>3. Eat with your fingers or a spoon. Sweet and crunchy!

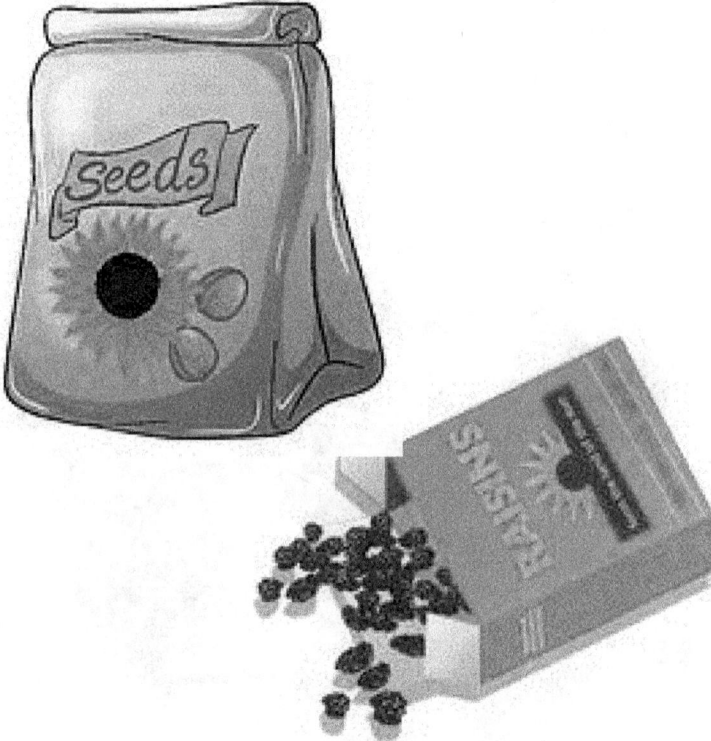

Honey Roasted Oats

Ingredients:
> Hot water
> ½ bowl of instant oatmeal
> Honey roasted peanuts
> 1 small pot, 1 bowl

Instructions:
> 1. In the pot, add water in the suggested amount given on the package and heat to a boil. Cook according to directions.
> 2. When the oatmeal is finished cooking, add the peanuts and stir.
> 3. Pour into a bowl and enjoy.

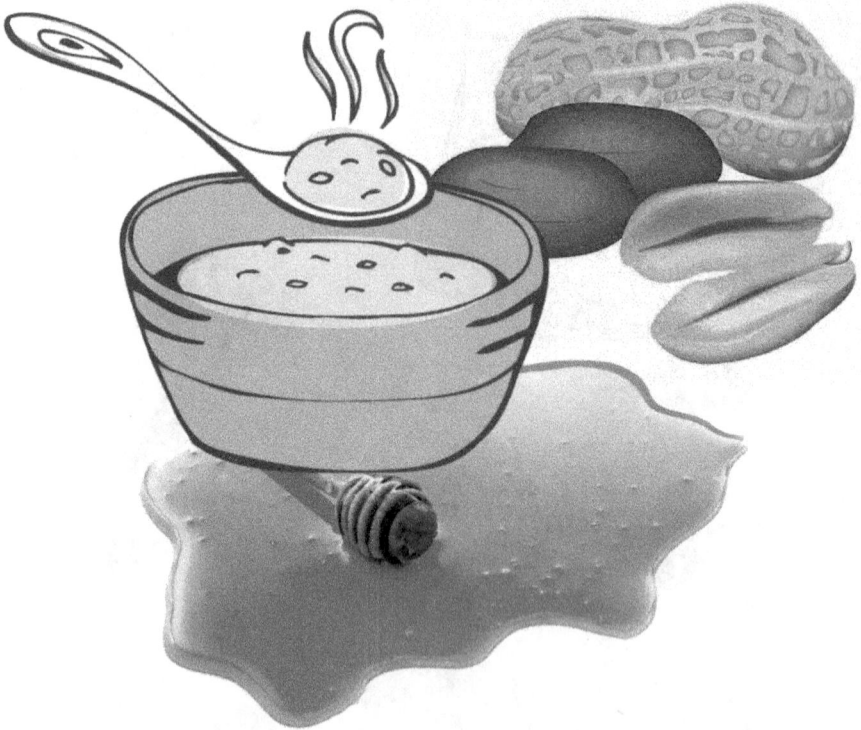

Chocolate Banana Pudding

Ingredients:
>   2 bananas
>   1 packet or 3 spoonfuls of sugar-free cocoa
>   1 bowl

Instructions:
1. Peel bananas and put them in the bowl. Smash them up with a spoon or use the peel as a barrier between your hand and the bananas.
2. Once fully smashed, dump the cocoa over the bananas and stir until the powder is completely dissolved and the mixture is smooth. Yummy!

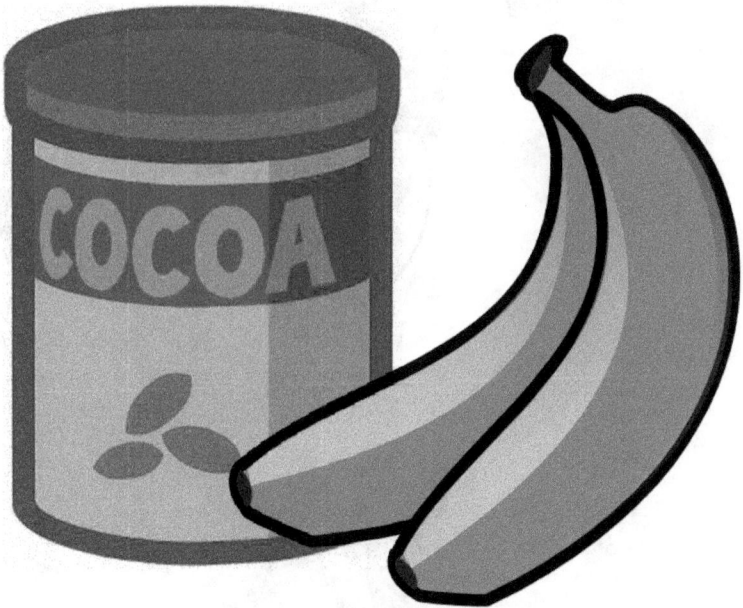

The All Natural

Ingredients:
>1 apple, sliced
>1 banana, sliced
>1 orange, in slices
>1 bowl

Instructions:
1. Put all the ingredients in the bowl and toss with your hand or a spoon
2. Eat a variety and enjoy!

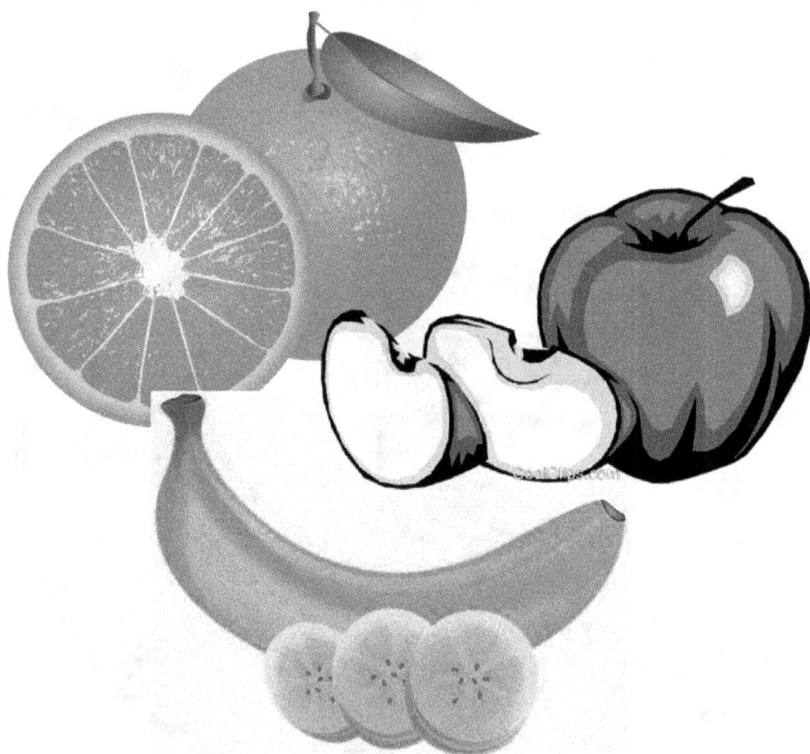

Sugar-Free Taffy

Ingredients:
>Hot water
>2 packs fruit punch Crystal Light, any brand
>½ bag of nondairy creamer powder
>1 bowl, 1 pair of latex gloves, 1 cup, 1 spoon

Instructions:
1. Pour creamer and Crystal Light into the bowl.
2. Fill the cup with hot water.
3. Using your spoon, get 3 spoonfuls of water out of the cup and pour over the mixture in the bowl.
4. Put on the gloves and start mixing the creamer mixture with the water.
5. After about a minute, there will be no more water to mix with the creamer. Add 2 spoonfuls of water and repeat.
6. Basically, you are going to start building a large clump. That clump is what you'll use to gather dry creamer when wet. When that clump can no longer gather any dry creamer because there is no more water, add 1-2 spoonfuls and start mixing and kneading until the clump is complete.
7. Be careful, too much water will ruin the taffy. Add more creamer if you accidentally overdo the water. If you don't have any more creamer, just start eating it. It will be very sticky. My favorite!

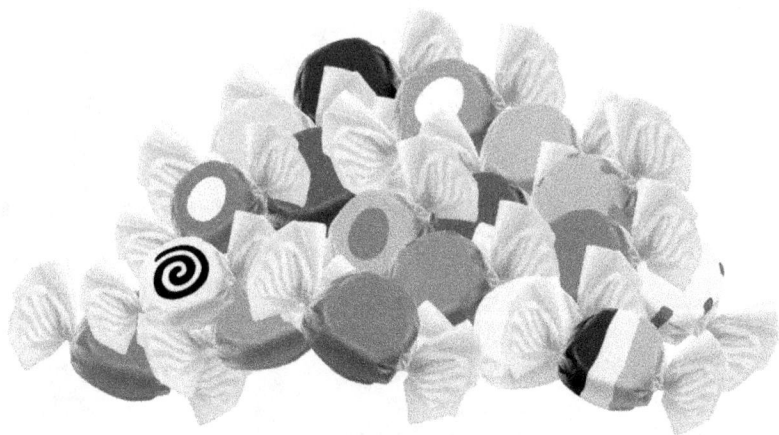

CHAPTER FOUR

"Chow Time, Chow Time!"

"If you can find a path with no obstacles, it probably doesn't lead anywhere."
– Frank A. Clark

You know you're on the right track when you encounter roadblocks and hurdles. People often give up when they are the closest to getting everything they've been working toward. Say the scale hasn't moved in two weeks, so you start eating your pastries again. In reality, your body was getting prepared to scorch fat, simply stabilizing itself before it got going. Nothing is going to be easy, and if it is, it's too good to be true. Break down those walls and clear those hurdles. You will be rewarded in the end.

Navigating the Chow Hall

This was a difficult part of the book to write because the menus are so different from state to state. I have compiled the menu items from ten states to find similarities that we all can use. I hope that you can find many similar menu items in your prison, but if not, you can at least get a basic idea of what you can use and what you can lose. Remember, all of our bodies react differently to food. You might find that you are able to eat a little extra than the recommendation, or you may find that you need to eliminate a little more than the recommendation in order to reach your weight loss goals If you keep these things in mind, I know you can do it!

I've created these recommendations from my experiences, along with many other people's experiences that showed results. My favorite part about these recommendations is that they still allow a taste of certain foods that you wouldn't expect. It is the same concept as many weight loss companies that claim, "Eat what you want and still lose weight!" That's because you're only eating a little bit of that pizza or cookie. Personally, I would wait until you are finished with the Carb Wean System and have figured out an intermittent fasting program that works for you before diving into these recommendations. This way, you can see some results and knock a few pounds off before you start treating yourself.

Without further ado, here are ideas for chow time.

Breakfasts

Pancakes

What's for Chow:	What to Eat:	Eliminate:
Pancakes x 4	1 pancake	3 pancakes
Oatmeal	Oatmeal	Butter
Egg	Egg	
Syrup		Syrup
Milk	Milk	
Butter (or Margarine)		Butter

Biscuits & Gravy

What's for Chow:	What to Eat:	Eliminate:
Biscuit	½ biscuit	½ biscuit
Creamed Beef	½ creamed beef	½ cr. Beef
Potatoes		Potatoes
Milk	Milk	
Cereal (Dry)		Cereal
Butter (or Margarine)		Butter

Breakfast English Muffin

What's for Chow:	What to Eat:	Eliminate:
English muffin	(Only eat ½	(½ of one &
Potatoes	of 1 of these)	all the other)
Ham	Ham	
Cheese	Cheese	
Cereal (dry)		Cereal
Milk	Milk	
Fruit	Fruit	

Tip: If ham is sliced, make wraps with the cheese; if ham is diced, shred the cheese into the ham.

Bacon & Eggs

What's for Chow:	What to Eat:	Eliminate:
Bacon	Bacon	
Scrambled eggs	Scrambled eggs	
Toast x4		Toast
Potatoes	½ potatoes	½ potatoes
Butter (or Margarine)		Butter
Milk	Milk	

Tip: Combine all the bacon, eggs and potatoes to make a scramble!

French Toast

What's for Chow:	What to Eat:	Eliminate:
French Toast x 4	1 slice	3 slices
Oatmeal	Oatmeal	
Syrup		Syrup
Milk	Milk	
Butter (or Margarine)		Butter

Waffles

What's for Chow:	What to Eat:	Eliminate:
Waffles x 2*	½ of one waffle	1 ½ waffles
Oatmeal	Oatmeal	
Syrup		Syrup
Milk	Milk	
Butter (or Margarine)		Butter

*If you get 3 or 4 waffles, eat 1 waffle since they will be smaller than 2 large waffles.

Beef Hash

What's for Chow:	What to Eat:	Eliminate:
Beef hash	½ beef hash	½ beef hash
Dry cereal		Cereal
Fruit	Fruit	
Milk	Milk	
Toast x 4		Toast
Butter (or Margarine)		Butter

Scrambled Eggs

What's for Chow:	What to Eat:	Eliminate:
Scrambled eggs	Scrambled eggs	
Cereal		Cereal
Fruit	Fruit	
Toast x 4	1 slice of toast	3 slices
Potatoes		Potatoes
Milk	Milk	
Butter (or Margarine)		Butter

Breakfast Burrito

What's for Chow:	What to Eat:	Eliminate:
Tortilla		Tortilla
Scrambled Eggs	Scrambled Eggs	
Cheese	Cheese	
Refried beans	Refried beans	
Salsa	Salsa	
Milk	Milk	

Tip: Either have the server put the cheese directly into the refried beans or do it yourself immediately. You will get the perfect melt!

Vegetable Scramble (eggs & cheese)

What's for Chow:	What to Eat:	Eliminate:
Vegetable Scramble	Vegetable scramble	
Hash browns		Hash brown
Oatmeal	Oatmeal	
Toast x 4	1 slice of toast	3 slices
Milk	Milk	

Pastry Day (cinnamon roll, apple fritter, coffee cake, etc.)

What's for Chow:	What to Eat:	Eliminate:
Pastry	½ pastry	½ pastry
Egg	Egg	
Cereal		Cereal
Fruit	Fruit	
Milk	Milk	

Lunches

Deli Sandwich (Any Meat)

What's for Chow:	What to Eat:	Eliminate:
Bread (slice or bun)		Bread
Deli meat	Deli meat	
Onion/pickle	Onion/pickle	
Chips		Chips
Lettuce	Lettuce	
Cheese	Cheese	
Veggies	Veggies	
Fruit	Fruit	
Mustard/Mayonnaise		Mayonnaise

Tip: Cut up meat and put into the veggies with your onions & pickles. Cut up cheese and put over the top. Add mustard and stir.

Fried Egg Sandwich

What's for Chow:	What to Eat:	Eliminate:
Bread x 2 slices		Bread
Fried Eggs	Fried Eggs	
Veggies	Veggies	
Mayonnaise		Mayonnaise
Cheese	Cheese	
Fruit	Fruit	

Tip: Cut up egg and cheese and put into veggies.

Hot Sandwich (any meat)

What's for Chow:	What to Eat:	Eliminate:
Bread x 2 slices		Bread
Meat	Meat	
Cheese	Cheese	
Mustard	Mustard	
Veggies	Veggies	
Fruit	Fruit	

Tip: Cut up the meat and cheese and put into the veggies.

Egg Salad Sandwich

What's for Chow:	What to Eat	Eliminate:
Eggs	Eggs	
Bread (slices or bun)		Bread
Mustard	Mustard	
Chips		Chips
Mayonnaise	Mayonnaise	
Veggies	Veggies	

Tip: If not done already by the kitchen, mix eggs into mayonnaise and mustard until fully blended. Eat it by itself or put it in your veggies.

Peanut Butter and Jelly Sandwich

What's for Chow:	What to Eat:	Eliminate:
Bread x 4 slices	1 slice bread	3 slices
Peanut butter	½ peanut butter	other ½
Jelly		Jelly
Veggies	Veggies	
Soup		Soup
Fruit	Fruit	

Tip: You can even go a step further and eliminate your 1 slice of bread and put the peanut butter on your fruit, preferably an apple or banana.

Fish Taco

What's for Chow:	What to Eat:	Eliminate:
Tortillas		Tortillas
Baked fish	Baked fish	
Rice	½ rice	½ rice
Veggies	Veggies	
Salsa	Salsa	
Fruit	Fruit	

Tip: Combine fish, rice and salsa into veggies.

Chef Salsa

What's for Chow:	What to Eat:	Eliminate:
Salad & Dressing	Salad & Dressing	
Ham	Ham	
Soup		Soup
Turkey	Turkey	
Eggs	Eggs	
Cheese	Cheese	
Breadstick	½ breadstick	½ breadstick
Fruit	Fruit	

Turkey Noodle Casserole (any casserole)

What's for Chow:	What to Eat:	Eliminate:
Turkey noodle casserole	Turkey	Noodles
Salad and dressing	Salad and dressing	
Bread (slices or dinner roll)	A small piece	Most of it
Veggies	Veggies	
Fruit	Fruit	

Tip: Put the meat from the casserole into the salad and dressing.

Hot Dogs

What's for Chow:	What to Eat:	Eliminate:
2 hot dog buns	1 hot dog bun	1 bun
2 hot dogs	2 hot dogs	
Catsup	Catsup	
Mustard	Mustard	
Veggies	Veggies	
Fruit	Fruit	

Tip: Put both hot dogs in one bun.

Grilled Cheese Sandwich

What's for Chow:	What to Eat:	Eliminate:
2 grilled cheese sandwiches	½ of 1 sandwich	1 ½
Tomato soup	Tomato soup	
Chips		Chips

Sunday Chicken or Pork Meal

What's for Chow:	What to Eat:	Eliminate:
Meat	Meat	
Macaroni salad		Macaroni
Salad and dressing	Salad and dressing	
Roll and butter		Roll & butter
Mashed potatoes		Potatoes
Veggies	Veggies	
Ice Cream	½ ice cream	½ ice cream

Tip: Make a meat salad!

Dinners

Pizza (any topping)

What's for Chow:	What to Eat:	Eliminate:
Pizza	Pizza toppings	Pizza crust
Salad	Salad (add pizza toppings)	
Soup		Soup
Dressing	Dressing	
2 Cookies	1 cookie	1 cookie
Chili		

What's for Chow:	What to Eat:	Eliminate:
Chili	½ chili	½ chili
Coleslaw	Coleslaw	
Baked potato		Potato
Brown rice	Brown Rice	
Cornbread	½ cornbread	½ cornbread
Butter		Butter

Meat Loaf

What's for Chow:	What to Eat:	Eliminate:
Meat loaf	Meat loaf	
Mashed potatoes		Potatoes
Hot veggies	Hot Veggies	
Gravy		Gravy
Bread slices	1 slice of bread	Rest bread

Cheeseburgers

What's for Chow:	What to Eat:	Eliminate:
Bun		Bun
Hamburger patty	Hamburger patty	
Cheese	Cheese	
Fries		Fries
Salad	Salad	
Dressing	Dressing	
Catsup/Mustard/Mayo	Catsup/Mustard/Mayo	

Tip: Mix meat and cheese into the salad!

Burritos

What's for Chow:	What to Eat:	Eliminate:
Tortillas	1 tortilla	All but 1
Refried beans	Refried beans	
Spanish rice	2 spoonfuls of rice	Rest rice
Shredded cheese	Shredded cheese	
Salsa	Salsa	
Salad	Salad	

Beef Stroganoff

What's for Chow:	What to Eat:	Eliminate:
Beef	Beef	
Noodles with sauce		Noodles
Salad	Salad	
Dressing	Dressing	
Bread		Bread
Vegetables	Vegetables	

Tip: Mix meat and salad for a tasty meal!

Spaghetti

What's for Chow:	What to Eat:	Eliminate:
Noodles		Noodles
Meat sauce	Meat sauce	
Vegetables	Vegetables	
Salad/Dressing	Salad/Dressing	
Bread		Bread

Tips: Put meat sauce over the veggies or on the salad. If your prison serves the noodles and sauce together, you can eat ⅓ of the spaghetti portion. Try to separate the noodles and sauce if you can though.

Macaroni & Cheese

What's for Chow:	What to Eat:	Eliminate:
Macaroni & cheese	⅓ Mac & cheese	⅔ Vegetable
Vegetables		
Bread		Bread
Fruit	Fruit	

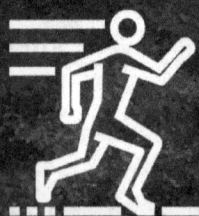

PART 3:
The Excercise Program

*"Excuses are the nails used to build
a house of failure."*
– Don Wilder

We all can come up with a ton of reasons why we didn't stick to the plan or go jogging this morning, but none of them are good. Showing up is the battle. Just do that, and everything else will fall into place. When it's yard line, put your exercise gear on and just show up to the yard, even on days when you're tired or full, whatever excuse you come up with today. Once you are out there in your gear, all that BS goes out the window, and you'll find yourself working out. Everyone has an excuse, and they all stink!

FOREWORD, PART 3

Your body is a tool of the mind; whatever your mind says to do, your body follows. Exercise is one of the rare times in which your body can challenge your mind and win!

It is a feeling like no other when your mind tells you that you can't run anymore and you keep going or that you can't do a push-up, and you do three more!

The mind is operating on a pain vs. pleasure system; the minute it feels pain, it will begin to tell you all of the reasons to get away from this pain. For example, running laps, your mind tells you, "Stop running before you pass out!" To add to this, your mind will send signals out so you actually *feel* like the message is true when in reality, no passing out is going to happen.

You will learn so much about yourself once you start exercising and moving around more. The wonders of the mind are truly amazing, and you'll really be surprised by what you find out about *yourself*!

This probably isn't your first time working out or stretching (although it could be), but this time you have a true workout partner in me. I will be with you every step of the way. I have been in your shoes at such a high personal weight that I felt it could never come down, or even if it did, the amount would be trivial. I was so wrong. Use these stretches and this workout to start knocking pounds down. It might take a short time; it may take a year or three years, so be it. Stick to the program. If you fall down, get back up again! You can do it! Whenever you need a pick-me-up, read this and get outside and exercise.

I believe in you!

Not My Favorite Thing

Now the fun begins. Exercise has never been my favorite thing to do. It still isn't, but I learned over a period of time that it is necessary for the weight loss goals I had in mind. Once I learned that I could send my calorie burning through the roof by exercising, I was all in. Eating right and drinking lots of water do the trick, but if there is a way to speed things up, I'm all for it.

Just knowing that I was only working out for calorie-burning purposes really took a lot of pressure off of me to lift heavy and burn myself out every day. I could actually take it easy, get my workout done in 30-40 minutes, and feel really good about it.

Going out to the basketball court, AKA the drama court, was no big deal for me because I told everyone repeatedly throughout the game, "I'm just trying to burn calories." Of course, I'd like to win, but calorie burning was my main objective.

Throughout the process, I never worried about results. I would just go outside every chance I had and do something. I knew that with my food choices, any workout would be beneficial. My mental health improved, my sleep improved, and I lost weight!

I would like to stress that stretching before and after workouts played a huge part, as my muscles really liked to tighten up. I have compiled most of the stretches and exercises I used and have trained others on, even my friends at the women's prison, and we all have had results. All in all, I have made exercise a major part in my life, which I now find it difficult to be without. I hope you enjoy

Getting Started

Starting a new routine of any kind can be a daunting thought on your mind. Exercise tends to rank in the top three routines that people often procrastinate about. We often provide ourselves with the reasons we can't begin an exercise program. We say to ourselves: "I don't want to be sore," "My fill-in-the-blank hurts," "I don't have time," or "The weather is bad," etc. None of these reasons makes any sense. You can literally find some sort of exercise that is easy on your body, that you can do inside, won't take much time, and will help you. Remember, the soreness you feel is your body getting stronger as it rebuilds itself.

We are on a weight loss journey, so this isn't a bodybuilding routine or anything of that nature. My favorite part of exercising to lose weight is that less is more. There is no need to lift heavy weights or do extreme cardio routines. The lighter the weight, the more repetitions you can do. A person may be able to lift only 150 pounds on the bench press three or four times, but the same person may be able to bench press the 45-pound bar by itself thirty or forty times! Those increased reps will burn far more fat than three reps of a higher weight. This is where you will shine!

Sitting on your bunk, thinking of exercising is not going to get you anywhere; believe me, I used to do this all the time. Put on your workout clothes and go to the place you plan to exercise. If you're walking or jogging, go to the track or do it in your cell; if you're doing push-ups, find a spot outside or do it in your cell. Once you show up at the *spot*, you've gotten the hardest part out of the way. Now all that you have left to do is do it! Today is the day. Just show up, and the rest will take care of itself.

"Trust yourself. You know more than you think you do." – Benjamin Spock, MD

If you think about it, you know a lot about weight loss and general health. Even at my heaviest of 276 pounds, I was more educated on health issues than the buffest guy on the yard. This was because I would read everything I could on weight loss and exercise that I could get my hands on. Now, whether or not I put that knowledge to use was a different story, but I had the information, nonetheless. I have a feeling you are the same way. Once I really decided to dedicate my time to losing 76 pounds, it seemed like everything I read and learned over the years began to come back. The same will happen to you. Trust and believe in you, and anything is possible!

CHAPTER ONE

Stretching

One thing we often neglect to do before and after a workout is stretch. Stretching allows our muscles, ligaments, and tendons to become more flexible, which is just as important as strength and endurance. The more flexible your muscles are, the less likely you are to suffer injury. Stretching also opens up muscles to better receive blood and oxygen. All of this allows for better movement and easier transition between workouts and day-to-day activities, as well as relieving many aches and pains.

Stretching when you first wake up in the morning is a great way to start your day for many reasons, such as the following:

- As you were sleeping, your muscles, joints, and ligaments tightened up. When you stretch, you loosen up all of your body as you stretch and make everything more flexible. You also help blood and oxygen flow as you stretch.
- Several minutes of stretching helps wake you up and puts you in a better mood that can last all day. Stretching releases endorphins in your brain, which are feel-good hormones, and we all could use more of those.
- You will also help your body start burning more calories when you stretch. By activating muscle groups in your body, your body will automatically need to find more energy. There will already be intense calorie burning going on while you were asleep, but stretching will be a boost to that burn. If you can avoid breakfast or any food until the afternoon, you will notice yourself losing weight after a while.

As you can see, stretching is an essential part of your physical, mental (and in some cultures) spiritual well-being. And best of all, it's free!

Foot & Ankle Stretches

Sitting Foot Rotations for Ankle Flexibility

- Sit on the edge of your bed or simply in a chair.
- Outstretch your left leg with toes pointed towards the floor.
- Sitting upright, start rotating your left foot clockwise 10 times.
- Bring your foot to a stop. Bring your left leg in.
- Repeat these steps with your right leg and foot, remembering to spin in a clockwise direction.
  Make sure to keep your leg still when rotating your foot.
- Stand up –Sit down.
- Repeat routine, but now rotate foot counterclockwise, one foot at a time.

Tip: Exhale upon rotation.

Standing Foot Rotations for Ankle Flexibility

- Stand upright, you can have a hand on a table or wall for balance.
- Lift your right foot off the ground and bring your right foot slightly backward until your toes are pointing straight down.
- Your foot should only be slightly off the floor. Do not strain yourself.
- Begin rotating your right foot clockwise with your toes pointed down 10 times.
- After the 10th rotation, rotate your right foot counterclockwise with your toes pointed down 10 times.
- Bring your foot back to the floor, placing it down flat.
- Repeat with your left foot.

Tip: Keep your opposite standing leg slightly bent while rotating your foot.

Toe Stretches

Toe Flex

- Sitting or standing, outstretch your legs and point your toes almost straight up into the air.
- Begin stretching and moving toes up, down, in, and out for 20 seconds.
- Once your toes are warmed up, clinch all your toes in and hold for 15 seconds.
- Relax your toes and outstretch them like you are reaching for something.
- Repeat this 5 times.

Toe Spread

- Sitting down, lift your right foot off the floor.
- Point your toes forward and slightly upward.
- Using the muscles in your toes, spread your toes as far apart as you can hold them for 5 seconds.
  Breathe deeply while doing this.
- Repeat this with your left foot.
- Do this 3 times with each foot.

Foot Stretches

Foot Nods

- Sitting down on your bed or in a chair, stretch both legs out with your toes pointed almost straight upward.
- Hold your legs in the same position the entire time.
- Slowly, using your ankle, bring your entire foot down until your toes are now pointing down.
- Now bring your toes back to pointing up.
- Repeat this motion for 1 minute.

Tip: Focus on keeping your toes straight while your feet nod.

Foot Windshield Wipers

- Sitting down, stretch both legs out with your toes pointed almost all the way upward.
- Begin moving your feet side to side, like windshield wipers.

- Go as far to the left and right as you can go, slowly.
- Each time you are fully stretched to either side, hold the position for 2 seconds each way.

Leg Stretches

Calves

Calves Stretch Rockers
- Standing up, using a table or wall for balance, go onto your tiptoes and hold for 5 seconds or more.
- Come back down flat-footed and rock back very slightly onto your heels, lifting only your toes off the ground.
- Come back to your tiptoe position and repeat.

If you battle with weight and are heavier, try the following:

- Stand facing a wall with your hands in front of you, palms facing the wall. Only stand about one foot or less away from the wall.
- Begin a slow fall towards the wall until you are on your tiptoes as your palms brace for impact.
- Push yourself back to the flat-footed position.

Tip: Do this slowly and breathe.

Calves Full Lunge Stretch
- Place both hands on the wall, shoulder width apart.
- Walk your feet back until your body is diagonal.
- Take your right leg and bring it towards the wall until your foot is flat and toes are almost touching the wall, and your left leg is still stretched behind you.
- Lean into the stretch and rock back and forth on your bent knee.
- Do this for 20 seconds.
- Bring your left leg in. Stand up straight and repeat using your other leg.

Hamstring

Raised Hamstring Stretch
- Find a flat surface to lift your right leg up on with your heel down on that flat surface.
- Use a stool, bed, table, etc., whatever height of a flat surface your flexibility allows you to use.

- Bend your weight-bearing leg slightly and try to reach for your toe on your right leg, which is in front of you, heel down on the flat surface. It will burn; that *is* the stretch.
- Do this for 15 seconds.
- Switch legs.

Lay Down Hamstring Stretch
- Lie down on your back.
- Put your feet down flat on the floor so your knees are bent, pointing towards the ceiling.
- Lift your right leg straight up so the bottom of your foot is facing the ceiling. If flexibility is a problem, just raise your leg as far upward as possible and hold.
- Feel the stretch in your hamstring.
- Hold your leg up for 15 seconds.
- Repeat twice, switching legs.

Tip: You can use a wall to help you hold your leg up. Lie down, lift your leg up straight into the air, and let your leg fall forward until your heel is resting on the wall. Hold for 15 seconds. Switch legs.

Thigh Stretches

Standing Thigh Stretch
- Stand up straight, arm's-length away from the wall.
- Put your left arm out with your palm facing the wall, then press your palm against the wall.
- Bring your right leg back behind you and lift your foot towards your buttocks until you can grab your ankle with your right hand.
- Using your left hand to brace yourself against the wall, hold your right ankle in your right hand for 15 seconds.
- Drop your leg back down to a standing position and switch legs.

Tip: If you can't grab your ankle behind your back, try this:

- Find a low, flat surface such as your desk stool or your bottom bunk (even your toilet will work if it's clean). Those at home can use a couch, love seat, etc.
- Turn your back on whatever your low surface is.

- Lift one leg behind you, raising your foot above the low surface; then let your foot slowly fall onto the flat surface so the top of your foot is resting there.
- This will stretch the same muscle until your flexibility gets better.

Knee Stretches

Knee Roll

- Stand up straight with your feet side by side, touching each other.
- Bend your knees slightly, then put your hands on each knee.
- Start making small circles with your knees as if you had a hula hoop around the top of your knees.
- Keeping your hands on your knees, make 10 circles in one direction and 10 circles in the other direction.

Tip: For even better stretching of the knee area during knee rolls, go slowly and alternate between small circles and wide circles.

Hip Stretches

Leg Turns

- Lie down on your back on a hard, flat surface.
- Put both feet flat on the floor so your knees are pointing upward.
- Put your left leg down flat. Keep your right leg in the same position as stated above.
- Place your hands on your stomach, palms down.
- Roll your left leg on your heel, inward and outward, so that your leg is rolling from left to right.
- On your outward roll, hold it at its outermost spot for 5 seconds.
- Do 15 rolls.
- Switch leg positions and repeat.

Squat Pause

- Stand with your feet a little bit wider than shoulder width. This means line up your feet, so they are a straight line up and down from your shoulders. Next, take a tiny sidestep outward past the shoulders.

- Bend your upper body slightly forward as if skiing downhill.
- Lower yourself into a squat and go as low as you can and *hold*.
- Stay in this position for 10 seconds.
- Come back up to a standing position. Shake out your legs.
- Repeat, each time trying to go lower than before.

Tip: Once you are comfortable with this stretch, try bouncing in very small pulses while holding the squat. Increase the time spent in this position from 10 seconds to 15, then 20, then 30. This will really open up your hips.

Back Stretches

Simple Low Back Stretch

- Lie on the floor or a hard, flat surface.
- Place your feet flat on the floor, so your knees are pointing upward.
- Focus on the lower back area and press it into the floor lightly.
- Interlock your hands and place your palms down on your stomach, keeping your neck straight.
- Tighten your stomach and really press your lower back into the floor.
- Hold this press for 10 seconds.
- Repeat 5 times.

Flipped Turtle

- Lie on your back with your feet flat on the floor so your knees point upward.
- Place your arms and hands at your sides on the floor with your palms down.
- Focus on the middle of your back and slightly press into the floor.
- Slowly start bringing your knees toward your chest as you focus on your middle back.

- If you can, as your knees are closest to your chest, grasp each of your back thighs (hamstrings) with each hand and pull closer to the body.
- Hold the stretch, with or without hands, for 20 seconds.

Tip: Try one leg at a time if this is too difficult.

Cat Back

- Get on your hands and knees. Keep your neck and back straight as you look at the floor in front of your hands.
- Take a deep breath in.
- As you breathe out, pull your stomach and chin toward your back until your back arches upward.
- You should be looking at your knees at this point.
- Hold this for 7 seconds.
- Return to the original position.
- Repeat 10 times.

Reverse Cat Back

- Get on your hands and knees. Keep your neck and back straight as you look at the floor in front of your hands.
- Take a deep breath in.
- As you breathe out, lower your stomach and raise your neck until your back has a dip in it and you are looking at the ceiling.
- Hold this for 7 seconds.
- Return to the original position.
- Repeat 10 times.

Still Jacks

- Stand straight up with your hands at your sides and your feet side by side.
- Slowly begin raising your arms to the sides until they are over your head, palms together like a jumping jack.
- Your feet do not move during this stretch.
- Once your palms are touching, hold for 5 seconds.
- Repeat 10 times.

Tip: Breathe in when raising your hands, breathe out when lowering your hands.

Sitting Twist

- Sit down on your bed or a chair with your back straight and looking forward with your knees forward.
- Cross your arms over your chest with one hand in your armpit and the other hand over your bicep.
- Take a deep breath in.
- Slowly and gently twist your upper body until you are looking over your shoulder. Keep your knees and feet facing forward. Hold for 3 seconds.
- Come back to the center.
- Now, again slowly and gently, twist your upper body until looking over the opposite shoulder you just did, and hold position for 3 seconds.
- Do this 5 times for each side.

Shoulder Stretches

Time-out Stretch

- Find a corner anywhere where two walls make a corner.
- Stand facing it like when we used to be in time-out. Stand one foot back.
- Place one hand on each side of the corner so you are touching two separate walls. You should look like you are about to do a standing push-up on the wall.
- Take a deep breath in.
- Slowly lean in and try to touch your nose to the corner, moving only your body, keeping your arms still.
- Feel the stretch in your shoulders.
- Hold for 10 seconds.
- Return to the original stance.
- Repeat 5 times.

Arm Rotations

- Sitting or standing, put both arms out like airplane wings. Your palms should be facing down, and your arms should be even with your shoulders.
- Have your knees and toes pointed forward and your face forward.
- Hold your arms there for 5 seconds.

- Make 10 very small circle-style rotations in a forward direction, like a bird flapping its wings, but in a circle.
- Now make 10 small circles in reverse.
- When you are done with that, drop your arms to your sides and shake them out.
- Bring your arms back up to shoulder height, palms down.
- Make 10 large circle-style rotations in a forward motion.
- Now make 10 large circles in reverse.
- Breathe evenly throughout.

Elbow Stretches

Elbow Hold

- Standing or sitting, reach your right hand in the air and then bring your hand down until your palm is touching your back, right under your neck.
- Your elbow should be pointing straight into the air.
- Using your left hand, palm your right elbow and press down gently.
- Hold this stretch for 10 seconds.
- Relax your arms and do it again, holding the opposite arm.

Wrist/Hand Stretches

Flat Table Stretch

- Standing upright, place both hands palm down on a table or desk or any raised, flat surface.
- Bend your knees slightly to lower into stance.
- Spread your hands as far away from each other as you can, keeping your elbows straight.
- Take a deep breath.
- Breathe out and keep your hands in place and elbows straight, lean your body weight over your hands. You want the weight on your wrists.
- Hold for 10 seconds.
- Lean back to the original position.
- Repeat 5 times.

Wrist Rounds

- Lightly ball both fists like The Rock when playing Rock-Paper-Scissors.
- From the wrist, rotate your fists in circles.
- Keep breathing steadily while rotating your wrists.
- Do 20 rotations in the same direction with both wrists, or one at a time.
- Switch directions and do 20 rotations.
- Outstretch your fingers until you are holding the #5 in each hand.
- Do wrist rotations 20 times in one direction with both wrists, or one at a time.
- Switch directions and do 20 rotations.

Tip: Do some rotations slowly and some fast for different results and a better overall stretch.

Clinches

- Outstretch your fingers until fully extended, including your thumb. Do this on both hands.
- Bring all your fingers and thumbs into your palm until a fist is made and squeeze.
- Hold this for 3 seconds.
- Breathe in and out slowly while squeezing.
- Release the squeeze and return your fingers to the original position.
- Do this 10-15 times.

Tip: Cut your fingernails to prevent any accidents.

Neck Stretches

Yes, Slow Nods

- Sitting or standing, look straight ahead.
- Slowly, only moving the neck, begin a slow nod towards the ground until you are looking at your feet.
- Hold for 4 seconds.
- Remember to breathe evenly.

- Now, using your neck only, begin a slow, upward part of the nod until you are looking straight up. Hold this for 4 seconds.
- Think of this as nodding *yes* in super slow motion.

No Slow Nods

- Sitting or standing, look straight ahead.
- Slowly, only moving your neck, turn your face to the right until you are looking over your right shoulder.
- Hold for 4 seconds.
- Remember to breathe evenly.
- Now, using your neck only, slowly start turning your face until you are looking over your left shoulder.
- Hold for 4 seconds.
- Think of this as saying *no* in slow motion.

Neck Rounds

- Sitting or standing, look straight ahead.
- Drop your chin all the way down by nodding your entire head downward.
- Going left using your neck, roll your head in a full circle, letting your head roll over your shoulder, back to your other shoulder, and back to the starting position.
- Breathe as you roll.
- Do 5 rolls going left.
- Repeat with 5 rolls going right.

Tip: Go slow and enjoy the pops.

Yoga Stretches

Plank

Start on your hands and knees. Tuck your toes under and straighten your legs back so your body comes into a push-up position. Keep elbows in line with wrist and avoid dropping hips. Extend forward through the top of your head. Hold for 60 seconds.

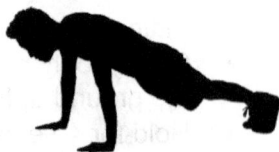

Down Dog

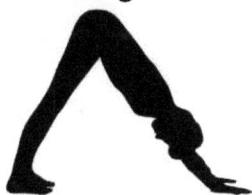

Lift your hips up and back to bring your body into an inverted V. Press your hands into the floor and your shoulders away from the floor. Relax your neck. Sway head side to side. Work toward pushing heels to the floor.

Down Dog Split

Keeping hips square and core engaged, raise your right leg up, foot bent, as high as you can. Avoid tensing muscles in your neck by pressing your shoulders away from the floor.

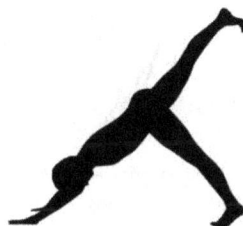

Knee-to-Elbow Crunch

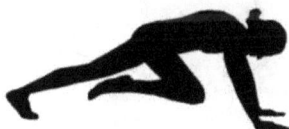

Rise up onto the toes of your left foot and lean your upper body forward. Bring the right knee to the left elbow, then the right elbow. Kick right leg back to Down Dog Split and hold.

High Lunge

Lift your hips up until the right thigh is parallel to the floor. Bring arms overhead, keeping biceps close to ears, fingers together. Breathe in deeply. If you like, sway your arms from side to side.

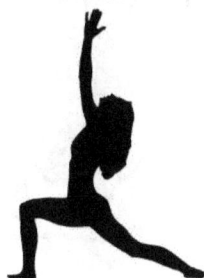

Revere Warrior

Turn left foot out to 45 degrees, bring heel to the floor. Lean back, sliding left arm down left leg to rest on thigh or calf. Reach your right hand toward the ceiling and look up.

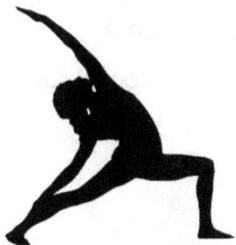

Upward Dog

Point your fingers to the top of the mat and hug your elbows in close to your ribcage. Inhale as you press

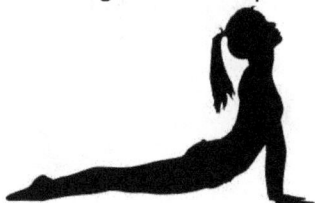

your hands firmly into the floor. Straighten your arms, lifting your torso and your legs a few inches off the floor.

Morning Yoga

Hold each pose for 10 seconds:

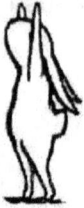 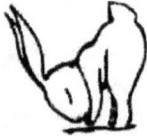 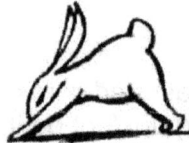 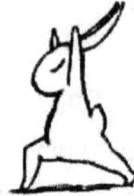

Mountain Pose   Forward Fold   Downward Dog   Warrior 1

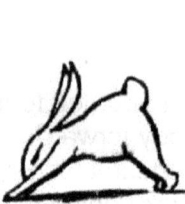 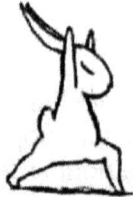 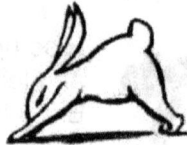 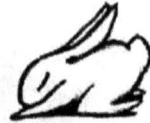

Downward Dog   Warrior 1   Downward Dog   Child's Pose

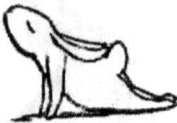 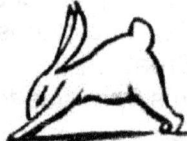 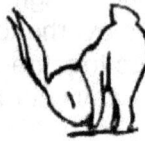 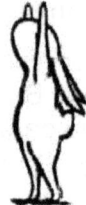

Upward Dog   Downward Dog   Forward Fold   Mountain Pose

Repeat this sequence six times every morning. Don't forget to breathe deeply and evenly, focus on your form, and keep your back straight.

CHAPTER TWO

Exercises

As we enter the exercise/workout portion of this book, I want to remind you to stay safe, stay hydrated, and stay focused. If you are just getting back into this or it's your first time working out, I'll be the first to let you know that it's no walk in the park, although you can choose that as an exercise. You are making the best decision of your life to give this a shot. You will be sore for days at times and feel parts of your body that you didn't even realize you had. Remember to stretch and drink lots of water.

Most of the workouts I listed can be done in a cell or anywhere, just make sure your cellmate is okay with it. If you are unable to do a workout, it is okay to improvise your own modified version.

The key is that you are active, and your heart rate is up past normal. As mentioned before, check with your medical provider before starting a new workout routine to make sure you are able to do what you want, and if not, you can adjust workouts to match the medical provider's recommendation.

Use the chart on the following page to understand how many calories you are burning during a workout. Remember, one pound of fat equals 3,500 calories. This means if you want to lose 1-2 pounds per week, you need to eat about 1,000 fewer calories every day, along with exercise. Yes, that seems small, but two pounds per week times 10 weeks equals 20 pounds! You got this!

Calories Burned by Exercise

Light Workout: Walking, Slow Cycling, Yoga

Your Weight (lbs.)	Calories Burned
130-169	4 cal./min. / 120 cal./30 min./ 240 cal./hr.
170-219	5 cal./min. / 150 cal./30 min. / 300 cal./hr.
220+	6 cal./min. / 180 cal./30 min. / 360 cal./hr.

Medium Workout: Walking Fast, Medium Cycling, Light Weight Training

Your Weight (lbs.)	Calories Burned
130-169	6 cal./min. / 180 cal./30 min. / 360 cal./hr.
170-219	7 cal./min. / 210 cal./30 min. / 420 cal./hr.
220+	8 cal./min. / 240 cal./30 min. / 480 cal./hr.

Intense Workout: Power Walking, Jogging, Heavy Weight Training, Sports

Your Weight (lbs.)	Calories Burned
130-169	9 cal./min. / 270 cal./30 min. / 540 cal./hr.
170-219	11 cal./min. / 330 cal./30 min. / 660 cal./hr.
220+	13 cal./min. / 390 cal./30 min. / 780cal./hr.

Use this chart to find out how many calories you burned during your workout today or to plan how many calories you'd like to burn.

The 30-Day Walk/Jog Challenge

If you go back and look at the Calories Burned Chart, you will notice something very awesome. If you jog a mile or walk a mile, you burn roughly the same number of calories!

We will use, for example, a 170-pound person. Let's say it takes 10 minutes to jog a mile in the Intense Workout box. It says that a person burns 11 calories per minute. Multiply that by 10 minutes of jogging. That equals 110 calories burned! If that same person walks a mile and this takes 25 minutes, according to the Light Workout box, it burns 5 calories per minute or 125 calories in that 25-minute period. Yes, the walking actually burned more calories, you see! How cool is that? It works this way for each box and column.

What this means for you is that you are either going to walk a mile or jog a mile each day for 30 days. You can even do it in your cell in laps or in place if you don't want to go outside.

Here is a walking chart so you can either count steps or count minutes to figure out when you reach your mile.

Distance	Walking Chart	
1/2 mile	1100 steps	12 1/2 minutes
1 mile	2200 steps	25 minutes
1-1/2 miles	3300 steps	37-1/2 minutes
2 miles	4400 steps	50 minutes

Low Impact Circuit Body Weight Exercises

Monday: #1 Basic Routine

Push-ups
- Get in the push-up position either on your hands and toes or hands and knees.
- Your hands should be shoulder-width apart (lined straight up and down with your shoulders).
- Lower yourself to the ground and push yourself up slowly back to the starting position.
- Do 5-10 push-ups.
- Take a 30-second break.

Squats
- Stand with your feet shoulder-width apart. Bend your knees slightly.
- Lean your upper body slightly forward.
- Bend your knees until your rear begins to touch the floor.
- Lift yourself back to having your knees in the slightly bent position.
- Do 5-10 squats.
- Take a 30-second break.

Dips (Beginner)
- Using a sturdy chair or bench, end of your bottom bunk bed, etc., sit down.
- Grasp the edge of the surface you are using with your palms facing down on top of the surface, fingers going down the front of the surface, and fingertips underneath.
- Push yourself up so your rear is off the seat. Maintain your hand grip.
- Inch your feet forward so your buttocks are in front of the seat.
- Your arms should be at a 90-degree angle as you dip your body towards the floor. Your buttocks will nearly touch the ground. Push yourself back up to the starting position.
- Do 5-10 dips.
- Start back at push-ups.
- Repeat 3 times.

Tuesday: #2 Cardio Basic

Walk/Jog 2 Laps
- Do one lap at a medium pace.
- Once you are back to the starting point, take a 30-second break.
- Now do another lap at a faster pace than above.
- Take a 30-second break.

Calf Raises
- Stand with your feet close together, but not touching.
- Raise yourself up onto your tiptoes.
- Lower yourself, almost letting your heels touch the floor.
- Raise yourself and lower yourself again.
- Do 20 calf raises.
- Take a 30-second break.

Air Traffic Controller
- Stand upright. Lift your arms up, even with your shoulders, palms facing each other.
- Move your arms out to your sides, like the wings of a plane, with your palms facing down.
- Raise your arms above your head until your palms are touching each other directly above your head. Your arms should be straight up.
- Bring your arms down to the starting position.
- Do this 10 times.
- Go back to the top, repeating this circuit 5 times, (Walk/Jog 2 Laps, Calf Raises & Air Traffic Controller).

Wednesday: #3 Build Up

Top of the Mornings
- Stand upright with feet shoulder-width apart.
- Put your hands behind your head with your elbows pointed outward, like relaxing in a lawn chair.
- Slightly bend your knees and keep your back straight as you take a bow.
- Keep your stomach tight.
- Slowly return to the starting position.
- Do 10-15 of these.

- Take a 30-second break.

Lunges

- Stand upright with your feet together and your hands at your sides.
- Take your right foot and step out as far as possible.
- Lower your left knee to the ground, bringing yourself as low as you can go.
- Push yourself back to the standing position by pushing up with your right leg.
- Now step out with your left leg, lower your right knee, and push up with your left leg.
- Do 5 lunges on each leg.
- Take a 30-second break.

Sidestep Squats

- Standing upright, take 2 side steps to the left as if moving out of someone's way.
- Do 2 squats. Stand upright.
- Take 2 side steps to the right.
- Do 2 squats. Stand upright.
- Do 10 squats in each direction.
- Go back to the top, repeating this circuit 5 times.

Thursday: #4 Flex Zone

Cherry Picking

- Stand upright with your feet wider than shoulder-width apart.
- Bend straight down to touch the floor. If you can't touch the floor, it's ok. Go as far as you can. Every time, try to go further than before.
- Keep your legs straight.
- From the middle, twist your body keeping your legs straight and feet forward, and touch your left toes (or as close as you can get).
- Come back to the middle and touch your right toes.
- Now, stand up straight.
- Repeat 10 times.
- Take a 30-second break.

High Climbers

- Using a raised surface or bar (even a wall), brace yourself with your hands on it.
- Walk your feet back until you are simply in a push-up position as you're standing.
- Keep your arms straight.
- Lift your right knee to your stomach and bring it back down.
- Lift your left knee to your stomach and bring it back down.
- Repeat this 15 times for each knee.
- Take a 30-second break.

Tip: Double count these, i.e., right knee, left knee equals one.

Standing Bicycles

- Stand upright, lifting your arms to shoulder height with your feet lined up with your shoulders.
- Lift your right knee up and touch it with your left hand. Return to normal position.
- Lift your left knee up and touch it with your right hand. Return to normal position.
- Do 20-25 of these exercises each and double count.
- Go back to the top, repeating this circuit 4 times.

Friday: #5 Full Circle Lite

- 5 Push-Ups
- 4 Squats
- 3 Dips
- Walk a Lap (or in place for 2 minutes)
- 5 Calf Raises
- 4 Air Traffic Controllers
- 3 Top of the Mornings
- Walk a Lap
- 5 Build Ups
- 4 Lunges
- 3 Sidestep Squats
- Walk a Lap
- 5 Cherry Pickings

- 4 High Climbers
- 3 Standing Bicycles
- Walk a Lap
- Go back to the top and do it one more time!

Medium Impact

Monday: #1 Twitch Fix

Hop Squats
- Stand upright with your hands in prayer position (palms touching and fingers upward).
- Bend your knees and lower your buttocks toward the floor.
- You should look like you are in the middle of a regular squat at this point. Hold.
- Now, hop just a little off the ground while holding the squat position.
- Do 15 hop squats.
- Take a 30-second break.

Push-up Jacks
- Get in the push-up position with your hands under your shoulders and feet close together.
- Do a push-up with your feet together.
- On the way up, spread your legs out so your feet are now far apart.
- Do a push-up with your feet out.
- On the way up, bring your feet back together.
- Repeat this 10 times, (5 close/5 wide).
- Take a 30-second break.

Jump Rope
- Jump rope for 30 seconds. (If your prison doesn't have jump ropes, just pretend.)
- Go back to the top, repeating this circuit 5 times.

Tuesday: #2 Cardio Go

Butt Kicks
- Begin by jogging in place for 5 seconds.

- Now bring your heels all the way up to the buttocks as fast (safely) as you can.
- Keep your arm swing controlled.
- Do this for 20 seconds.
- Take a 30-second break.

Regular Crunch

- Lie on your back, bringing your knees up toward your chest with toes pointed out.
- Place your hands around the back of your head with your elbows pointing toward your knees.
- Bring your elbows and knees together, flexing your stomach as you do.
- Separate your knees and elbows, relax your stomach, and repeat.
- Do 10-30 of these. If you can't get to 10, do as many as you can until you reach 10.
- Take a 30-second break.

Knee Ups

- Begin by jogging for 5 seconds.
- Now bring your knees all the way to your chest as fast (safely) as you can.
- Keep your body upright and arm swing controlled.
- Do this for 20 seconds.
- Go back to the top, repeating this circuit 5 times.

Wednesday: #3 Core Power

Bar Raisers

- Standing upright, lift your arms up and in front of you at shoulder height with palms down.
- Slowly bring your right knee up to your right arm.
- Now bring your left knee up to your left arm quickly as you bring your right leg back down.
- Keep switching your legs.
- Do this for 20 seconds.
- Take a 30-second break.

Plank

- Get into the push-up position with your hands under your shoulders and feet close together.

- Your arms should be straight as you are all the up. Keep your back straight.
- Hold this position for 30 seconds or more.
- You will notice yourself lowering to the ground. Push yourself back up. Enjoy the shaking!
- Take a 30-second break.

Bar Dips
- Use a dip bar or 2 even surfaces.
- Grasp each bar or surface with each hand and push yourself up so your feet are off the floor. Keep your arms straight.
- Bend your elbows slowly to lower yourself closer to the bar/surface. Breathe in.
- Push yourself back up to the straight arm position. Breathe out as you do.
- Repeat this 5-10 times.
- Go back to the top, repeating this circuit 7 times.

Thursday #4: Full Body

Slow Burpee
- Standing upright, bring yourself slowly into the push-up position.
- Do a single push-up.
- Now, bring yourself back up to standing.
- Repeat 5 times.
- Take a 30-second break.

Ski Slope Hop
- Bring yourself into the squat position with your hands lightly balled up next to your hips.
- Do a side jump, keeping yourself facing forward, and thrust your fists behind you like you are skiing.
- In your new position, bring your fists back to the side of your hips.
- Now, side jump back to the starting point, doing the same hand motion.
- Do 10 of these.
- Take a 30-second break.

Low Plank
- Get into the push-up position. Instead of using your hands to hold yourself up, lower yourself onto your forearms to hold yourself up.
- Keep your back flat.
- Hold this for 30 seconds or more.

Friday #5: Full Circle Medium

- 5 Hop Squats
- 4 Push-up Jacks
- 15 Second Jump Rope
- Walk/Jog a Lap
- 15 Second Butt Kick
- 10-20 Crunches
- 15 Knee Ups
- 45-second break
- 15-second Bar Raisers
- 20-second Plank
- 5 Bar Dips
- Walk/Jog a Lap
- 3 Slow Burpees
- 6 Ski Slope Hops (3 each side)
- 20-second Low Plank
- Walk/Jog a Lap
- 45-second to 1-minute break
- Go back to the top and do everything 1 more time, all the way down!

High/Intense Impact Circuit

Monday #1 Cross Circuit

Regular Burpees
- Stand straight up.
- Bring yourself into a squat.
- Place both hands on the ground, palms down, while still in a squat.
- Spring your feet back until you are in the push-up position.

- Do a push-up.
- Bring your feet back underneath your body as you push up.
- Stand straight up.
- Do this 10 times.
- Take a 20 second break.

Do 15 Jump Squats
- Do a regular squat and jump on the way up.
- Take no break.

Jog a Lap
- Take a 1-minute break.
- Do this 10 times.

Tuesday #2 Bear Down

- Do 5 Burpees
- On the 5th Burpee, after your push-up, stay in the push-up position.
- Do a 10-foot Bear Crawl. If you're in a cell, go up and down until 10 feet.
- Walk like a bear on your hands and feet.
- Walk half a lap.
- Jog the other half.
- Take a 1-minute break.
- Do this 10 times.

Wednesday #3 Plyo Flex

- Do 5 Regular Burpees.
- Then do 5 Jump Burpees, where instead of simply standing, jump in the air as high as you can.
- Do this 10 times.

Thursday #4 Full Plyo

- Do a Plyo Push-up where, on the way up, push your body up hard so your hands come off the ground, bend elbows slightly while in the air to cushion the landing.
- Do 7 of these.

Plyo Squat/Lunges

- Get in the squat position, jump up, and land in a deep squat.
- Jump up in the air again and land in a lunge with your right leg forward.
- From that lunge, jump up and switch legs, landing with your left leg forward.
- Jump up from that lunge and land in a deep squat.
- Squat – jump – lunge – jump right – lunge – jump left equals 1.
- Do 8-10 of these.
- Starting from the top, do this 10 times.

Friday #5 The Tap Out

- Do 50 Regular Burpees in sets of 10.
- Do 1 Bear Crawl for 10 feet.
- Do 25 Jump Burpees in sets of 5.
- Take a 2-minute break.
- Repeat one more time.

*"Everywhere is within walking distance
if you have the time."*
– Steven Wright

You can and will do it all once you start, as long as you don't let anything or anyone stop your progress. It might be a slower process than you'd care for, but positive things will be happening regardless. Nothing is beyond your reach as long as you are making choices every day to reach it.

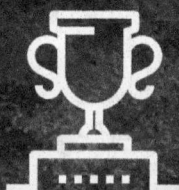

PART 4:
More Motivation

*"Everything comes to he
who hustles while he waits."*
– Thomas Edison

This is something that is not to be taken lightly. The outcomes that you want in life await you, but as you push yourself towards these results, there is a substantial stagnant period as your actions produce results. In those in-between times, do a little extra work to supercharge your outcomes. Practice being kind to someone you don't really like. Share with someone in need (within the rules). Work to become a better person, a better family member, a better friend, while you wait for your health journey to pay off. Whatever you know you need to work on, work on that, and at the end of this, you will be the best you've ever been.

"Well done is better than well said."
– Benjamin Franklin

So many times I talk about all the things I want to do when I get out, but I make little to no effort to even educate myself on what I need to do to accomplish it. One example is an App for phones and tablets, I think would make me at least a "hundred thousandaire," but I haven't looked into coding, app design, or even programming. There are even companies that can do all of the work for me, and I haven't even looked into that. We all do this, especially in our health journey. Let's change our ways and start making an effort to turn our dreams into reality.

*"Determine that the thing can and shall be
done, and then we shall find the way."*
– Abraham Lincoln

Determination is what separates the talkers from the doers. Setting the goal and action plan is vital to accomplishing anything, but putting your words into action takes sheer determination and drive. I know when I was eating poorly, and I had two servings of cake, nothing was going to stop me from finishing my main course and both cakes, no matter how full I became. Using that same determination on the opposite end of the spectrum can be beneficial. Nothing can stop me from eating right or exercising now, and you definitely have the same determination within yourself.

"All glory comes from daring to begin."
– Eugene F. Ware

To start anything meaningful can be nerve-racking because none of us wants to fail. You can be assured that after the first time, your endeavors will get easier and each time after that. The key is to *do it*. You'll never know if you don't try.

"Life is like a dog sled team. If you ain't the lead dog, the scenery never changes."
– Lewis Grizzard

Get out in front of the situation by ignoring everything that can hold you back. You know your triggers; mine is homemade / commissary cheesecake. Not only do I avoid the entire section on the commissary sheet where the ingredients are sold, but I also avoid the people on my unit who make these delicious cakes. If I don't, I'll be stuck in my old ways at my old weight. Therefore, I have formed my own lane in which I'm the leader of my own destiny. If you want to work out every day, you can't hang out with people who are going to hold you back from doing that. It's a hard pill to swallow, but your health is more important than anything because without your health, you have nothing.

"What great thing would you attempt if you knew you could not fail?"
– Robert H. Schuller

Putting limits on ourselves is a learned behavior. It's time to shed that learning and start living your life without limits. When it comes to how many pounds you would like to lose or how many laps you would like to run, nothing can stop you from doing something every day to get closer to achieving that. You will not fail if you keep at it each day. Let others tell you that you can't, and then prove them wrong.

> *"Go the extra mile. It's never crowded."*
> *– Executive Speechwriter Newsletter*

The bare minimum isn't good enough! You can get what you want faster and build confidence and self-esteem by pushing yourself just a little past what you thought was your breaking point. It can be quite lonely, and you'll learn a lot about yourself, plus you will appreciate the journey even more. Not many people have the drive that you do, and that's why you can go harder and farther than they. Now go get it.

> *"The person who goes alone can start today, but he who travels with another must wait until the other is ready."*
> *– Henry David Thoreau*

Although many people won't do anything unless they have a partner, and there are benefits to having a workout or diet partner, the real results are going to come when you do your own thing. You never know when your workout partner might need to take a few days off for illness, injury, or just plain laziness. You also don't know what your dieting partner is doing late at night (when you're asleep) with that box of Honey Buns.

These first steps need to be yours and yours alone. Once you figure out how you operate and where your strengths and weaknesses lie, you can find a partner whose goals are aligned with yours or even someone who can help you. By doing it solo, you'll learn more about yourself than you thought you did, and you'll have no one to blame for your success but yourself.

"The best vision is insight."
– Malcolm S. Forbes

Take a look inside yourself today. See how all of the good things and things that you perceive as bad that have happened in your life have all worked together to make you who you are today. During good times and bad, we don't always realize that everything is working to make us stronger and better.

Looking within, seeing the changes that have taken place and the changes that are to come, you get an opportunity to grow and learn. Nobody can take this from you!

"Not until we are lost do we begin to understand ourselves.
– Henry David Thoreau

Finding your way is the hardest thing you can do. It is within this struggle that makes you who you are and pushes you past your limits. Beginning healthy nutritional habits can make you feel as if you are lost in the wilderness, but the beauty of it all is that as you begin to navigate your path back to the path you want to be on, you will learn what works perfectly for you. That is a priceless gift you can give to yourself.

"You may find the worst enemy or best friend in yourself."
– English Proverb

Sometimes, looking in the mirror can be a mind-blowing experience. The person looking back is what you created. Positive self-talk and affirmations can help you not become your worst enemy. Nobody else will love you (or hate you) like you do, so try with everything you have to love yourself, compliment yourself, and believe in yourself. With that, you will start becoming your own best friend, the best friend you've ever had.

Paul J.R. Dawson

"Often, we change jobs, friends, and spouses instead of ourselves."
– Akbarali H. Jetha

It's always easier to point the finger and blame everyone and everything for our problems. To say, "If it wasn't for them, I wouldn't be in this situation," not only helps us justify our actions but relieves us of any responsibility for the situation. The hard part comes when we look internally and force ourselves to say, "If I didn't put myself in that situation, then I wouldn't have this issue."

Take the time to think of the things you blame others for. Challenge yourself to see what your role was in the situation and if you have any ownership in it. I used to blame the prison for serving so much bread and unhealthy items, but it is *my* choice how much of it I eat and whether I eat it at all. Yes, it will suck. But owning a situation gives you all of the power back and an opportunity to fix it and make things better. Try it!

"Argue for your limitations and, sure enough they're yours."
– Richard Bach

What you decide that you can do will be what you do. Limitations are only in your mind. I found out when doing push-ups that if my goal was 20 push-ups, I would start losing energy at around 17 or 18, but if I said I wanted to do 30 instead, even after a few sets of 20, I wouldn't start losing energy until 27 or 28. It worked for every workout. I learned quickly how to trick my mind into surpassing my limitations. Simply telling yourself, "I got this," or "C'mon, you can do it," will let your mind know that it's *go time* and you can exceed your wildest expectations. Argue for better progress, never limitations.

*"Self-respect is the fruit of discipline;
the sense of dignity grows with
the ability to say no to oneself.*
– Abraham Joshua Heschel

Saying no is very hard. We all want to help or share, especially with those we are close to. It takes practice and will tear you up sometimes, but it must be done. What about saying no to yourself? On chocolate chip cookie night, can you say no? Can you say no to eating the bread at lunch when you are hungry? Once you begin to say no to yourself, your power grows. Getting your self-control under control is not easy, but it must be done.

*"The better we feel about ourselves,
the fewer times we have to knock
somebody else down to feel tall.*
– Odetta

Don't forget what you learned in elementary school. The mean thing a person says about someone else is really how that person feels about himself. Happy people don't even bother to bring others down. If anyone is discouraging you from reaching your goals, it is because they have already been discouraged from their own goals. Successful people want to see others succeed. Once, a skinny person called me fat; I later found out that they had been trying to gain weight unsuccessfully for years. This revelation was proof that looks can be deceiving, and even though the person bringing you down might appear to have it all together, remember they wouldn't be bringing you down if they truly had everything down pat. Don't go to their level. Keep pushing yourself to reach your goals. You might even motivate them and others around you to start seriously pursuing their goals!

"Nothing happens unless first a dream."
– Carl Sandburg

Everything you see around you all started with a thought or a dream. The inventor could have let his idea be a fleeting thought or told his friends that he had a crazy dream and gone into detail, but instead, he took action. Whatever you see around you came from a person taking action on their dream. What is your weight loss dream? Take action *today*!

> *"The best way to make your dreams come true is to wake up."*
> *– J.M. Power*

I can daydream all day about my goals, but I know that none of it will become a reality without putting forth some sort of effort. At times, certain things may seem crazy or unobtainable, such as a six-pack of abs, but if that is your dream, start trying. Even if you don't get to the six-pack, with effort and dedication, you'll one day have a flat stomach and feel better about yourself than you did when you started.

Wake up from that dream and start making power moves towards reaching that dream. It's yours for the taking!

> *"Discipline is remembering what you want."*
> *– David Campbell*

It can be confusing while working towards a distant goal. Often, distractions, pessimism, and unforeseen hurdles come out of nowhere and try their best to derail our dreams. There is a positive side to these things happening – they serve as reminders that you are on the right track! If you were not on the right track, you would not encounter these attempted derailments. Keep telling yourself what you are working for and why. These reminders will keep you focused and help you find tons of solutions to any obstacle that foolishly tries to stand in your way.

> *"Don't bunt. Aim out of the ballpark."*
> *– David Ogilvy*

Go for it all! Even if your goal seems lofty, go for it. The amazing thing is that you do have the possibility of achieving the goal, and at least you will come close. Instead of trying to lose 100 pounds, aim to lose 150 pounds. Instead of aiming to run one mile, aim for two. Even if you don't get the full two miles, the first mile will seem like nothing.

"A rock pile ceases to be a rock pile
the moment a single man contemplates it,
bearing within him the image of a cathedral.
– Antoine de Saint-Exupery

Weight loss is no longer a struggle, the minute you begin to see it as a fun and life-changing experience. Make everything in your life positive because you can control how you interpret any and all situations. Simply changing your thinking can make something enjoyable that you once would have never considered to bring you joy.

"Dreams and dedication are
a powerful combination."
– William Longgood

Changing your own ways is only going to be as hard as you make it. When it comes to your eating, you already have the dream or idea of where you want to be; now is the time to dedicate to that. When you fuse your idea with a dedicated work ethic, you will be unstoppable!

"Whoever wants to reach a distant goal
must take many small steps.
– Helmut Schmidt

Short-term goals are going to be your best friend while you travel on this weight-loss journey. It would be great if we could lose all the weight we wanted in two weeks, but that is not going to happen. A reasonable short-term goal can be something like 3-5 pounds a week. It doesn't sound like much, but it will add up. In four weeks, that's 12-20 pounds! If your goal is 100 pounds of weight loss, that will take 20-33 weeks. Small steps toward a big goal will keep you motivated and most importantly help you actually complete the goal!

> ### *"When you aim for perfection, you discover it's a moving target."*
> *– George Fisher*

There are so many different people telling us what we should be striving to look like, and none of them are right. You could spend years trying to look like someone else's version of perfect, and once you finally get there, their definition changes. I've seen women spend their whole lives trying to become as skinny as possible because the magazines and movies essentially say, "Skinny is perfect." Then, once she is skinny, here come the Kardashians, so now the "perfect body" is not skinny, according to those same magazines and movies.

My message is, don't aim for perfection, especially someone else's version. Go for what will make you comfortable and happy.

> ### *"There is nothing worse than being a doer with nothing to do."*
> *– Elizabeth Layton*

Assess your surroundings to make sure what you are setting out to do is actually doable in your current environment. Everywhere has pros and cons that can either aid us or prevent us from reaching our goals. Write down your goals and then make sure that you have the resources to complete them.

*"The hardest thing to learn in life to learn
is which bridge to cross and which to burn."*
– Laurence J. Peter

Changing habits can be challenging. While switching from
purchasing pastries and cookies to peanuts and pork rinds was
truly difficult, it was well worth it. Yes, the fear of missing out and
the sight of everyone else eating the things you view as
delicious will be a delicate practice in willpower, but you will
soon realize that by leaving certain foods out of your life, you will
improve your life tremendously.

*"Think big thoughts
but relish small pleasures."*
– H. Jackson Brown, Jr.

It is easy to get caught up in the hustle and bustle of reaching
your goals. There is a certain mindset of people when they get
focused. It reminds me of a laser-locked missile, almost robotic.
In that frame of mind, we usually forget to take the time to stop
and smell the roses.

Simply take a few minutes each day and just remind yourself of
all the things you are grateful for. It will make the journey even
more rewarding and help you navigate your day to reach your
goal with a smile on your face.

*"The truth of the matter is that you always
know the right thing to do.
The hard part is doing it."*
– General H. Norman Schwarzkopf

Sometimes the hardest thing to do is the right thing. That's why
it's the right thing. But once you do it, it's done, and you can
walk away knowing that you did the right thing. You know now to
avoid that bread and that cake. Walk past it, give it away, or

don't buy it at the store. Yes, it will be hard, but well worth it, and you *can* do it.

> ## *"Self-discipline is when your conscience tells you to do something and you don't talk back."*
> *– W.K. Hope*

How you respond to a situation is all that matters. Just because Jim offers you a candy bar doesn't mean you have to accept it. The best way to learn self-discipline is to start learning how to say no: "No, I can't accept that. No, I'm not making spreads anymore." Soon it will become a habit, and you'll have disciplined yourself.

> ## *"How old would you be if you didn't know how old you were?"*
> *– Satchel Paige*

There is a time for seriousness, but not all the time. Continue to find the child within and let go of all the pressures that can weigh you down at times. You are only as old as you feel, so try to feel like you did when you were younger, and you didn't have a care in the world except having fun!

> ## *"Great opportunities to help others seldom come, but small ones surround us every day."*
> *– Sandy Koch*

Little things matter. Just saying hi to a person or helping them pick up something they dropped can change a person's day or life. One thing to keep in mind is this: what you do will be passed on/paid forward. Although what you do may not seem significant, it is.

"Character consists of what you do on the third and fourth tries."
– James Michener

Rarely do we get it right the first time. Microsoft wasn't Bill Gates' first company. Michael Jordan wasn't a top basketball player in high school and barely made the team. The true magic happens when you pick yourself up and try again, each time becoming better than you were before. This creates character and will strengthen you as a person.

"You can measure someone by the opposition it takes to discourage them."
– Robert C. Savage

There will always be somebody trying to throw you off your game. They might be doing it intentionally or unintentionally. Either way, it doesn't matter because you have the drive within you to overcome any obstacle in your way. It may be jaw-dropping at times to see the new ways some people will come up with to thwart your endeavors, but just remember, it falls into the same category, opposition. The only thing that matters is your triumph over the opposition as you get back to reaching your goal.

"How a person plays the game shows something of their character, how they lose shows all of it."
– Tribune (Camden County, GA)

You never know how your plans will turn out. We all want to win, but there are no guarantees. Even when things don't go your way, take it as a learning experience and a win. Sometimes when you lose, you'll find out later that you really win.

"The reputation of a thousand years may be determined by the conduct of one hour."
– Japanese Proverb

We know that better than most due to being incarcerated, but the key is not to let your crime define you. I know that after my sentence, I let it carry me into a pit of despair, and I gained nearly 80 pounds over time. Once I remembered who I was, who I am, and who I could be, I was ready to lose those pounds. You can do it too; just look within!

"An optimist stays up until midnight to see the new year in. A pessimist stays up to make sure the old one leaves."
– Bill Vaughan

Perception can never lose. What you see and feel about any situation is the "truth" to you, and anybody who disagrees with you can "shut the front door," so to speak, right? Knowing that, your job is to train your brain to see things as positively as you can. When the scale goes up, a positive note from that can be, "Okay, I guess I can't sneak in those pancakes," or "Maybe I can push myself a little harder during cardio." Think positively. Be an optimist, and things will always be up.

"If you don't want anyone to know, don't do it." *– Chinese Proverb*

What's done in the dark *will* come to the light. Sneaking in a Pop-Tart and a bag of chips *will* slow down and/or reverse your weight loss goals. This journey of health is one in which your efforts are either rewarded or hindered based on what you do when nobody is looking. Make sure not to hold yourself back because you deserve to reach your full potential.

"When there is an original sound in the world, it wakens one hundred echoes."
– John A. Shedd

You'll inspire others on your health journey in ways you can't even imagine. Some will want to know how you did it so they can emulate you. Others will think, "If he can reach his goals, then I can reach my goals too." How cool is that?

"Nothing valuable can be lost by taking time."
– Abraham Lincoln

Effort is everything, and the more time you put into perfecting your goals, the better your results will be. You will be able to find the best direction for you and how to maximize your outcomes. Putting in the time is all that counts; everything else will fall into place after that.

"Be patient with everyone, but above all yourself."
– St. Francis de Sales

You are your own *worst* critic, but it is time to become your own *best* critic, just like your artist friend who draws a beautiful piece of artwork but points out all the flaws that nobody else would've noticed otherwise. That is what you do to yourself. Instead, start pointing out all the good things and give yourself credit. It will not happen overnight, so be patient with yourself and your goals.

"Courage is being scared to death and saddling up anyway."
– John Wayne

I've always admired the courage of First Responders, knowing the bomb went off, the house is on fire, etc., and still running into the fray. That is how you can look at your weight-loss journey. Just like those First Responders, you can save a life, a very important life, *yours*! Run into this situation with courage, no matter how scary or daunting it may seem. You will come out on top!

"Facing it, always facing it, that's the way to get through. Face it." – *Joseph Conrad*

Hiding from your problems doesn't help anyone. It allows the problem to go unchecked and grow bigger until it builds up too high. The minute you address the problem, you stop it at its growing point; it has no choice but to shrink. You can't control much, but you can confront any problem in your life with confidence and courage.

"Fall seven times, stand up eight."
– Japanese Proverb

Time and time again, adversity pops its head up to let you know that things might get a little crazy. Adversity will push you and knock you down. It's all good, though, because you are much more of a fighter than adversity is, and all you have to do is shake it off, get up, and get back to what you were striving for. Adversity will never give up, and neither should you.

"By perseverance, the snail reached the Ark."
– Charles Haddon Spurgeon

We are all at different stages in our weight loss journey. Some of us are in pretty good shape and would just like to lose ten pounds or less. Others of us are in bad shape, where our life is in danger, needing to lose 150 pounds or more. Whichever the case, you are in control and have to lock your mind on getting to where you want to be. It might be slow, but it will be well worth it.

"Don't tell me how hard you work. Tell me how much you get done."
– James Ling

Actions have always been louder than words. We all have that friend that *tells* us all about their diet and exercise plan and how perfect they are at it. But we constantly *see* them eating things they claim to never eat and missing workouts. Well, talk is cheap. Get to work and start earning your results so you can get to where you want to be.

"There are no shortcuts to any place worth going."
– Beverly Sills

If you really want this, you are going to have to go the distance and grind it out. Taking the easy way doesn't let you appreciate what you've been through and how you got there. Just like a 16-year-old who gets a Mercedes for their first car probably won't appreciate it like a 60-year-old who worked their whole life for the same car. When you take short-cuts, you cut yourself short. The struggle is real but so are you. You can get there the right way.

"Good habits are as easy to form as bad ones."
– Tim McCarver

Twenty-one days is the average amount of time it takes the human brain to form a neural pathway of habit. Lying in bed all day for 21 days will become a habit just as easily as waking up at 6:30 each morning and doing 50 push-ups for 21 days. Your job is to start forming good habits to replace your bad habits, and 21 days is all you need. Start today.

> *"Nothing great was ever achieved*
> *without enthusiasm."*
> *– Ralph Waldo Emerson*

You are on a mission, a mission to get healthier. Some days will not be as exciting as others, but you can always remind yourself to be excited for yourself and the mission you are on. Put a smile on your face and some pep in your step, even if you aren't feeling that way, and watch what happens. Before you know it, you'll be feeling great, excited about your mission again, and ready to take on the day!

> *"Dig the well before you are thirsty."*
> *– Chinese Proverb*

Planning is one of the keys to success. The good thing about you is that you are smart and have all the tools to plan the perfect strategy to lose weight. Looking at the menu the day before to see what you can eat and what you need to pass up is huge. Avoiding certain areas on the commissary sheet and talking to the people you know who are cooking all the time can help you execute your plans down to a science. You can always change your plans until you find the perfect one for you, but having a plan to start with is crucial. Take time today and write down five goals you want to get done this week regarding eating and exercise, then work each day to accomplish each one.

> *"Not everything that is faced*
> *can be changed. But nothing can be*
> *changed until it is faced."*
> *– James Baldwin*

I still remember the day I realized that I had to write a book to share this weight loss program with people in custody. I know some people will do almost everything they read, while others will do almost everything they can to avoid doing any of the plans I have laid out. The beauty of this is that you are in full control once you have the information. Face the issue and change your life.

> *"These things are good in little measure and evil in large: yeast, salt and hesitation."*
> *– The Talmud*

Pace yourself during this health journey; you don't want to overexert yourself to the point that you experience burnout. Remember, everything in moderation, and you will ensure yourself an energy level and drive that you might find surprising!

> *"The reward for work well done is the opportunity to do more."*
> *– Jonas Salk, M.D.*

As you mark boxes off your goal chart, set new ones. Maybe your goal was to walk 2 miles a day for 6 months. Now go for 3 miles. Push yourself to do better, and you will. This journey will need to become a lifestyle eventually, and you never want to become complacent or revert back to late-night cookies just because you lost 40 pounds. Always strive for more, and then *do* more.

APPENDIX:
DOC Fat and Calorie Guide

Item	Serving Size	Calories	Fat
Beverages			
Chow Hall			
Coffee	single serving	0	0
Tea	single serving	0	0
Fruit Drink	8 ounces	0	0
Skim Milk	16 ounces	160	0.5
Canteen			
Carnation Breakfast drink	1 packet	130	0.5
Cocoa/Creamer/Milk			
Creamer	1 teaspoon	10	0.5
French Vanilla Cappuccino	3 tablespoons	100	3.5
French Vanilla Creamer	4 teaspoons	60	2.5
Hot cocoa w/marshmallows	3 tablespoons	190	15
Nestle whipper mix	3 tablespoons	120	3
Powdered nonfat milk	1/3 cup	80	0
SM no sugar added cocoa	1 envelope	60	
Vanilla Caramel - sugar free	1 tablespoon	30	2.5
Coffee			
BC Decaf	1 rounded teaspoon	4	0
Columbian FE	1 rounded teaspoon	4	0
Expresso FE	1 rounded teaspoon	4	0

Maxwell house	1 rounded teaspoon	4	0
Tasters choice	1 rounded teaspoon	4	0
Crystal light			
Fruit Punch	2/5 packet	5	0
Iced Tea	2/5 packet	5	0
Lemonade	2/5 packet	5	0
Orange	2/5 packet	5	0
Peach Tea	2/5 packet	5	0
Raspberry Ice	2/5 packet	5	0
Raspberry lemonade	2/5 packet	5	0
Drink mixes			
Country Time Lemon/Berry			
Gatorade Fruit Drink	1 2/3 tablespoon	80	0
Mandarin/Tangerine	11/2 tablespoon	90	0
Sweet Tea with Lemon	1 1/2 tablespoon	90	0
Tang	2 tablespoons	100	0
Watermelon Strawberry Kool-Aid	2 tablespoons	90	0
Welch's Grape Juice	1 bottle	180	0
Powdered nonfat milk	1/3 cup	80	0
Tea			
Bromley Decaf Tea Bags	1 bag	0	0
Celestial Seasonings Tea	1 bag	0	0
Golden Tip Tea Bags	1 bag	0	0
Green Tea - Bigelow	1 bag	0	0
Vending Machine			
A&W Cream Soda	20 ounces	290	0
A&W Diet Root Beer	20 ounces	0	0
Lipton Green Tea	20 ounces	120	0
Mountain Dew	20 ounces	290	0
Mountain Dew Code Red	20 ounces	290	0
Sunkist Orange	20 ounces	270	0

Pepsi	20 ounces	250	0
Pepsi Wild Cherry	20 ounces	260	0
Ruby Red Squirt	20 ounces	280	0
Multi Movie			
Coke	20 ounces	240	0
Diet Dr. Pepper	20 ounces	0	0
Dr. Pepper	20 ounces	250	0
Minute Maid Cran-Grape	15 ounces	1	0
Bread Products			
Chow Hall			
Bagel	1 each	240	1
Biscuit (Large)	1 each	225	2
Biscuit	2 each	280	1.5
Bread Stick (2 ounce)	1 each	180	3
Bun	1 each	240	2
Cornbread	1 each	250	6
Dinner Roll	2ea	280	1
Flour Tortilla	1 each	100	4
Flour Tortilla	2 each	200	8
French Bread (2 ounce)	1 serving	170	2
French Bread Toast	2 slices	460	4
French Toast	2 slices	460	8
Grilled Bread	2 slices	220	2
Grilled Bread	4 slices	440	4
Grilled Wheat Bread	2 slices	221	2
Grilled Whole Wheat Bread	2 slices	210	2
Hamburger Bun	1 each	240	2
Hoagie Bun	1 each	240	2
Multi-Grain Bread	2 slices	160	2
Wheat Dinner Rolls	2 each	280	1
Wheat Hoagie Bun	1 each	240	2

Wheat Tortillas	1 each	100	2
Whole Wheat Bread	2 slices	160	2
Whole Wheat Bread	4 slices	320	4
Whole Wheat Toast	2 slices	160	2
Texas Toast	2 slices	460	4
Toast	2 slices	160	2
Canteen			
Plain Bagel	1	280	1
Tortillas 8"- Cactus Annie's	1	110	2.5
Chi Chi's White Corn Tortillas	2	120	1.5

Breakfast cereals

Chow Hall			
Oatmeal	10 oz.	185	3
Nine Grain Cereal	10 oz.	160	1
Farina	10 oz.	140	1
Dry Cereal	10 oz.	220	1
Canteen			
Cinnamon Squares	3/4 cup	130	3
Dry Bulk Oatmeal	1 ounce dry	150	3
Frosted Flakes	3/4 cup	120	0
Frosted Mini Wheats	1 cup	180	
Granola Cereal - Fruit & Nut	2/3 cup	240	7
Mom Raisin Bran	8 ounces	220	1.5
Fruit/Cream Oatmeal			
Bananas & Cream	1 packet 35g	130	2
Blueberries & Cream	1 packet 35g	120	2
Peaches & Cream	1 packet 35g	130	2
Strawberries & Cream	1 packet 35g	130	2
Variety Oatmeal			
Apple and Cinnamon	1 packet 35g	130	1.5
Cinnamon and Spice	1 packet 35g	160	2

Maple and Brown Sugar	1 packet 35g	160	2
Raisin and Spice	1 packet 35g	150	1.5

Cakes, pastries, etc.

Chow Hall			
Bagel	1 each	250	1.5
Bread Pudding	4 ounces	155	3.5
Breakfast Pastry	1 each	350	25
Baker's Choice	1 serving	300	3-15
Bar Cookie	1 each	255	3-10
Carrot Cupcake	1 each	250	10
Frosted Cupcake	1 each	250	10
Fruit Cobber	1 each	350	8
Fruit Crisp	1 serving	180	8
Chocolate Brownie	1 each	340	8
Pudding	4 ounces	150	3.5
Pudding - Chocolate	4 ounces	150	4
Pudding - Butterscotch	4 ounces	120	2
Pudding - Vanilla	4 ounces	140	3.5
Pudding - Banana	4 ounces	130	2.5
Pudding - Lemon	4 ounces	120	2
Pumpkin Bar	1 each	250	13
Canteen			
Apple Pie - Miss Freshley's	1	470	27
Cherry Pie - Miss Freshley's	1	480	27

Candy, chocolate

Canteen			
Atomic Fireballs	3	60	0
Butterfinger	1 bar	250	10
Certs - Peppermint	1 mint	0	0
Certs - Wintergreen	1 mint	0	0
Fast Break Candy Bar	1 bar	230	11

Gracey's Butterscotch Disc	3 pieces	60	0
Gracey's Starlight Mints	3 pieces	60	0
Hershey's Candy Bar	1 bar	210	13
Hershey's Candy Bar w/Almonds	1 bar	210	14
Jellybeans	14 pieces	160	0
Jolly Rancher - Assorted	3 pieces	70	0
Jovy Revolcaditas Candies	1	25	0
Lemonheads Bag	10 pieces	50	0
Licorice Twist - Black	4 Twist	140	0
Licorice Twist - Red	4 Twist	140	0
M & M Plain	1 bag	230	9
M & M Peanut	1 bag	250	13
Milky Way	1 bar	240	9
Orange Slice – E.Z. Digby's	3 pieces	140	0
Orange Slice Candles – Sathers	3 pieces	140	0
Reese's Peanut Butter Cup	1 package	210	13
Snickers Candy Bar	1 bar	250	12
Snickers with Almonds	1 bar	230	9
Sugar Free – Wild Fruit	4 pieces	45	0
Sweet Obsession Chocolate Bar	8 pieces	200	11
Sweet Obsession w/Peanuts	8 pieces	210	13
Three Musketeers Candy Bar	1 bar	240	7
Twix Candy Bar	2 cookies	250	12
Vanilla Caramels	7 pieces	190	4
Multi Movie			
Junior Mints	16 pieces	170	3
Sugar babies	28 pieces	160	1.5
Hot Tamales	20 pieces	140	o
Cheese Products			
Chow Hall			
Cheese	1/2 ounce	50	3

Cheese	1 slice	60	4
Cheese - grilled cheese sandwich	4 slices	240	16
Cheese Sauce	2 ounces	120	3
Shredded Cheese	1 ounce	100	5
Canteen			
Cheese Bar - Cheddar	1" cube	90	7
Cheese Spread -Habanero	1 ounce	90	8
Cheese Squeeze - Jalapeno	1 ounce	90	8
Cheese Squeeze - Cheddar	1 ounce	90	9
Hot Pepper Cheese	1" cube	90	7
Mozzarella Cheese	1" cube	90	7
## Chicken			
Chow Hall			
BBQ Chicken	4 ounces	190	12
Breaded Chicken Pattie	1 each	240	12
Baked Chicken Quarter	1 each	250	12
Chicken	3 ounces	150	12
Chicken A la King	6 ounces	185	25
Chicken Baked Quarter	1 each	250	12
Chicken Filling	3 ounces	150	12
Chicken Frank	2 each	270	24
Chicken Fried Steak	1 each	285	12
Chicken Kielbasa	1 each	260	24
Chicken Patti	1 each	240	12
Chicken Salad	4 ounces	210	14
Southern Chicken	1 each	160	12
Teriyaki Chicken	4 ounces	190	12
Premium Chicken Breast Filling	4.5 ounces	112	2.5
BC Chicken Taco	1 pouch	480	
## Chips			
Chow Hall			

Cheetos Oven baked	1 bag	120	4.5
Chips	1 bag	150	9
Lay's Potato Chips	1 bag	160	10
Rold Gold Pretzels	1 bag	110	1
Sun Chips - Harvest Cheddar	1 bag	140	6
Tortilla Chips	2 ounces	280	16
Canteen			
Chili Cheese Fritos	1 bag	320	19
Cool Ranch Doritos	1 bag	260	13
Cracklins w/Hot Sauce	.5 ounce	80	6
Flaming Hot Cheetos	1 bag	320	22
Jalapeno - Miss Vickie's	1 bag	210	12
Lay's Cheddar/Pepper	1 bag	200	11
Mini Pretzels	17 pieces	110	1
Nacho - Cactus Annie's	1 ounce	150	8
Nacho Cheese Doritos	11 chips	140	9
Original Cheetos	1 bag	310	21
Original Fritos	1 bag	320	20
Pork Rinds	.5 ounce	80	5
Rounds - Cactus Annie's	11 chips	140	6
Ruffles Cheddar Sour Cream	1 bag	130	4
Condiments			
Chow Hall			
BBQ Sauce	1 ounce	25	0
Catsup	1 ounce	30	0
Catsup	1 tablespoon	15	0
Margarine	#60 scoop	90	5
Mayonnaise	1 tablespoon	50	4.5
Mustard	1 tablespoon	10	0
Salsa	2 ounces	15	5
Canteen			

BBQ Sauce	2 tablespoons	60	0
Cactus Annie's Medium Salsa	2 tablespoons	10	0
Chili-Garlic Sauce	1 teaspoon	0	0
Cinnamon	1teaspoon	15	0
Garlic Powder	1 tablespoon	28	0
Green Chili Sauce	1 ounce	10	0
Mayonnaise packets	1 packet	50	4.5
Mustard	1 tablespoon	0	0
Panola Soy Sauce	11	0	1
San Miguel Salsa Verde	60g	30	1
Siam sauce	1 tablespoon	35	0
Tabasco Squeeze packet		0	0
Tapatio Hot Sauce	1 teaspoon	0	0
Cookies			
Chow Hall			
Cookie	1 serving	300	9
Bar Cookie	1 each	255	3-10
Pumpkin Bar	1 each	250	13
Lemon Bar	1 serving	250	6
Caramel cookie bars	1 cookie	170	8
Chocolate Cream Cookies	3 cookies	150	6
Coconut Macaroons	1 cookie	210	13
Duplex Cookies	3 cookies	150	5
Keebler Chocolate Chip Cookies	2 cookies	153	29
Oreo Cookies	1 package	250	10
Peanut Butter Cream Cookies	3 cookies	150	6
Strawberry Creme Cookies	3 cookies	150	6
Strawberry Fig Bar	1 bar	70	1
Vanilla Cream Cookies	3 cookies	150	5
Crackers			
Canteen			

Chicken Cracker	10 crackers	150	8
Keebler Club Crackers	4 crackers	70	3
Ritz Crackers w/ peanut Butter	1 pack	200	11
Saltine Crackers	5 crackers	60	1.5
Snack Crackers	5 crackers	80	4
Wheat Crackers	16 crackers	130	3.5

Cream and creamers

Canteen

Creamer	1 teaspoon	10	0.5
French Vanilla Creamer	4 teaspoons	60	2.5
Vanilla Caramel - sugar free	1 tablespoon	30	2.5

Desserts

Chow Hall

Brownie	1 serving	340	8
Cookie	1 serving	300	9
Frosted Cupcake	1 each	250	10
Fruit Cup	1 serving	180	0
Lemon Bar	1 serving	250	6
Peach Crisp	1 serving	180	8
Pudding	4 ounces	150	3.5
Pudding - Banana	4 ounces	120	2.5
Pudding - Butterscotch	4 ounces	130	3.5
Pudding - Chocolate	4 ounces	190	6
Pudding - Lemon	4 ounces	120	2.5
Pudding - Vanilla	4 ounces	140	3.5

Eggs, egg dishes

Chow Hall

Cheese Omelet	1 each	200	16
Egg Patty	1 each	90	5
Egg Salad	4 ounces	175	7
Fried Egg	1 each	90	5

Fried Eggs – breakfast	2 each	165	10
Fried Eggs – sandwich	2 each	180	10
Fried Egg – Breakfast sandwich	1 each	90	5
Fried/Scrambled Eggs	2 each	165	10
Hard Boil Egg	1 each	70	5
Scrambled Eggs	3 ounces	135	7
Scrambled Eggs - Hobo Breakfast	2 ounces	88	4.5
Vegetable Cheese/Scramble	4 ounces	180	5
Vegetable Frittata/Scramble	4 ounces	180	5
Canteen			
Ovaeasy Whole Egg	2 tablespoons.	70	5

Margarine, mayonnaise

Chow Hall			
Garlic Butter	#60 scoop	90	5
Margarine	#60 scoop	90	5
Mayonnaise	1 tablespoon	50	4.5
Mustard	1 tablespoon	10	0
Canteen			
Mayonnaise	1 tablespoon.	50	4.5

Fish

Chow Hall			
Salmon Pattie	1 each.	240	18
Baked Fish Filet	3 ounces	135	12
Canteen			
Tuna	4.23 ounces	110	0.5
Mackerel	1/3 cup	70	2

Fruit, fresh, dried

Chow Hall			
Apple	1 each	55	0
Peach	1 each	60	0
Canned Fruit	1 each	60	0

Fresh Fruit	1 each	90	0
Grapefruit Half	1 each	60	0
Orange	1 each	45	0
Pear	1 each	75	0
Banana	1 each	65	0
Canteen			
Demonte Prunes	1-1/2	100	0
Kars Banana Chips	1 ounce	150	9
Sun Maid Raisins	2 ounces	120	0
Ice cream			
Chow Hall			
Bowl – Neapolitan	1 scoop	130	6
Good Humor Vanilla Sandwich	1 each	130	2.5
Canteen			
Chocolate Peanut Butter	4 ounces	170	9
Cookie Dough	4 ounces	160	8
Cookies and Cream	4 ounces	150	7
Ol' South Fudge	4 ounces	150	7
Tin Roof	4 ounces	150	8
Vanilla	4 ounces	130	7
Vending Machine			
Cookie and Cream Sandwich	1	250	10
Heath Ice cream Bar	1	290	0
Vanilla – Ice Cream Sandwich	1	20	7
Mississippi Mud – Sandwich	1	280	9
Entrees and sides			
Chow Hall			
Beans	6 ounces	180	1
Beef Potato Casserole	10 ounces	375	11
Beef Stroganoff	6 ounces	250	19
Chicken & Broccoli Casserole	10 ounces	300	11

Chicken & Rice Casserole	10 ounces	425	19
Chicken Ala King	6 ounces	185	25
Chicken Enchilada Casserole	10 ounces	530	24
Chili Mac	10 ounces	350	11
Ham Au gratin	10 ounces	375	15
Ham & Bean Stew	10 ounces	300	11
Hearty Beef Stew	10 ounces	280	11
Hobo Breakfast	1 serving	263	13.5
Italian Casserole	10 ounces	375	15
Macaroni & Cheese	10 ounces	450	14
Ranch Style Chili	10 ounces	350	20
Ranch Style Beans	10 ounces	300	13
Tamale Pie	10 ounces	400	24
Turkey A la King	6 ounces	190	25
Turkey Noodle Casserole	10 ounces	350	14
Turkey Tetrazzini	10 ounces	355	23
White Bean Chicken Chili	10 ounces	280	2
Canteen			
Breakfast Bowl	1 bowl	39Q	22
Chili – Back Country	1 packet	290	6
Instant Chili	1/2 cup	220	4
Hot Refried Beans & Rice	1 cup	460	5
Meat			
Chow Hall			
Bacon	3 slices	135	12
Baked Pork Loin	3 ounces	165	12
BBQ Beef	3 ounces	180	12
BBQ Beef	4 ounces	240	16
BBQ Pork Loin	3 ounces	200	12
Beef Filling	3 ounces	220	12
Beef Hash	8 ounces	320	14

Beef Patty	1 each	225	12
Beef Sausage Patty	2 ounces	160	8
Beef Spread	4 ounces	180	16
Beef Stroganoff	6 ounces	250	19
Bologna	3 ounces	180	24
Creamed Beef	6 ounces	235	12
Deli Meat	3 ounces	150	24
Ground Beef	1 ounce	75	4
Ham	2 ounces	110	8
Ham Scramble	3 ounces	200	16
Hot Dogs	2	280	48
Meatloaf	5 ounces	285	16
Pig in Blanket	2	440	48
Pork - Fajita	3 ounces	195	12
Roast Beef	3 ounces	180	12
Roast Beef	3 ounces	180	12
Roast Beef w/Salsa	4 ounces	190	12
Roast Pork Loin	3 ounces	180	12
Salami	3 ounces	270	24
Salisbury Steak	1 serving	300	15
Sausage Gravy	6 ounces	265	12
Seasoned Beef	3 ounces	225	12
Sliced ham	3 ounces	180	12
Sloppy Joe	4 ounces	250	12
Taco Meat	3 ounces	210	12
Tuna Salad	4 ounces	160	12
Canteen			
BC Chorizo	1 pouch	600	33
Beef Barbacoa		170	0
Carnitas Pork	3 ounces	250	15
Hot & Spicy Sausage	2 ounces	160	13

Paul J.R. Dawson

Oberto Cocktail Pep Bites	2 ounces	200	17
Oberto Original Beef Jerky	1 ounce	50	3
Oberto Peppered Beef Jerky	1 ounce	80	1
Oberto Teriyaki Beef Jerky	1 ounce	80	1
Pepperoni Stix	1 stick	170	13
Spam Classic	1 package	250	22
Summer Sausage	2 ounces	160	13

Nuts, seeds, nut butters

Chow Hall			
Peanut Butter – Breakfast	1.5 ounce	252	21
Peanut Butter – Lunch	2.5 ounce	420	35
Canteen			
Banana Chips	1 ounce	150	9
Cashews	1 ounce	152	14
Corn Nuts - BBQ	1 pack	180	6
Honey Roasted Peanuts	1 ounce	165	14
Hot Peanuts	1 ounce	107	5
Mixed Nuts	1 ounce	170	15
Natural Almonds	1 ounce	160	
Peanut Butter – chucky	2 tablespoons	200	16
Peanut Butter – creamy	2 tablespoons	200	16
Salted Peanuts	1 ounce	310	25
Sunflower Kernels	1 ounce	166	15
Unsalted Peanuts	2 ounces	200	17
Whole Enchilada Mix	1 ounce	140	9

Pancakes and waffles

Chow Hall			
Pancakes	4 each	340	30
Waffles	3 each	300	3

Pasta, noodles

Chow Hall			

Weight Loss Unlocked

Pasta Salad	6 ounces	200	1
Pasta	6 ounces	160	1
Parsley Pasta	6 ounces	155	1
Spaghetti Noodles	6 ounces	166	1
Canteen			
Beef	1/2 block	190	7
Cajun Chicken	1/2 block	190	7
Chicken	1/2 block	190	7
Chili	1/2 block	190	7
Hot & Spicy Vegetable	1/2 block	190	7
Texas Beef	1f2 block	190	7
Thai Chili Noodle	1 pack	780	12

Pies

Canteen			
Apple Pie - Miss Freshley's	1	470	27
Cherry Pie - Miss Freshley's	1	480	27

Poultry

Roast Turkey	3 ounces	135	9
Sliced Turkey	3 ounces	120	9
Turkey	1 ounce	35	3
Turkey	3 ounces	120	9
Turkey – chef salad	1 ounce	35	1.5
Turkey Bacon	3 slices	120	4
Turkey Ham – Chef Salad	1 ounce	35	1.5
Turkey Ham – Breakfast Sandwich	1 ounce	35	1.5
Turkey Ham – deli	2 ounces	70	3
Turkey Salami	3 ounces	180	14

Pizza

Chow Hall			
Pizza – Choice	1 serving	525	24
Pepperoni Pizza	1 serving	525	24

Vending machine			
Red Baron Pepperoni	1	420	20
Red Baron Supreme	1	410	19

Rice and Rice Dishes

Chow Hall			
Brown Rice	6 ounces	160	1
Brown Rice Pilaf	6 ounces	180	5
Spanish Rice	6 ounces	180	4.5
Steamed Rice	6 ounces	155	0
Canteen			
Hometown Spanish Rice	4 ounces	170	1.5
Hot Refried Beans & Rice	1 pouch	460	5
Rice – Brown	4 ounces	140	1
Rice – White	4 ounces	160	0

Salads

Chow Hall			
Beet Salad	6 ounces	100	0
Cabbage Salad	6 ounces	115	0
Chicken Salad	4 ounces	210	15
Coleslaw	6 ounces	110	0
Cowboy Salad	4 ounces	100	0
Gelatin Salad	6 ounces	125	0
Gelatin Salad w/whip topping	4 ounces	100	2
Garden Salad	10 ounces	20	0
Garden Vegetable Salad	6 ounces	30	0
Green Salad	10 ounces	15	0
Lettuce Salad	10 ounces	10	0
Macaroni Salad	6 ounces	210	7
Marinated Veg Salad	6 ounces	80	0
Mixed Greens	10 ounces	15	0
Pasta Salad (without/with mayo)	6 ounces	200	1/7

Potato Salad	6 ounces	225	10
Texas Slaw	6 ounces	100	8
Tossed Salad	10 ounces	10	0
Tuna Salad	4 ounces	160	12
Egg Salad	4 ounces	175	15

Salad Dressing

Chow Hall			
1000 Island	2 ounces	240	11
French Dressing	2 ounces	260	25
Ranch Dressing	1 ounce	120	16
Vinaigrette	1 ounce	90	9

Sauces and gravy

Chow Hall			
Chicken Marinara	6 ounces	300	6
Chicken Gravy	2 ounces	50	4
Creamed Beef	6 ounces	235	12
Cream Gravy	2 ounces	50	4
Cream Sauce	2 ounces	50	4
Dill Sauce	2 ounces	80	4
Gravy	2 ounces	50	4
Marinara Sauce	4 ounces	60	3
Meat Sauce	6 ounces	300	4
Sausage Gravy	6 ounces	265	12
Soy Sauce	1 ounce	20	0
Tartar Sauce	1 ounce	70	7
Turkey Gravy	2 ounces	50	4
Canteen			
Tapatio Hot Sauce	1 teaspoon	0	0
Chili Garlic Sauce	1 teaspoon	0	0

Seasonings and spices

Chow Hall			

Soy Sauce	1 ounce	20	0
Salsa	2 ounces	15	0
Canteen			
Jalapeno Wheels	1	5	3
Yellow Chili Peppers	.7 ounces	5	0

Snacks, popcorn, chips

Canteen			
Blueberry Cheese Danish	1 Danish	480	22
Buttered Popcorn	1 ounce	160	10
Little Debbie's donut sticks	1 donut	230	14
Fudge Brownies		280	12
Fudge Dip Granola Bars	1 bar	150	7
Honey Buns		230	13
Nutty Bar Cookies	2 cakes	310	18
Oatmeal Creme Pies		170	7
Microwave Popcorn			
Kettle Corn		31	16
Lite Butter		50	5
Extra Butter		30	11
Pop Tart			
Strawberry	1 pastry	200	5
Wild Berry	1 pastry	200	5
Chocolate Fudge	1 pastry	200	5
Raspberry Cereal Bars	1 bar	150	3.5
Strawberry Cheese Danish	1 Danish	470	21
Swiss Cakes Rolls	2 cakes	270	12
White Cheddar Popcorn	1 ounce	170	12

Soups

Chow Hall			
Egg Flower Soup	10 ounces	80	2
French Onion Soup	10 ounces	100	1

Lentil Soup	10 ounces	150	9
Onion Soup	10 ounces	90	0
Potato Soup	10 ounces	180	7
Soup of the Day	10 ounces	150	9
Tomato Soup	10 ounces	105	1
Vegetable Chowder	10 ounces	150	8
Vegetable Soup	10 ounces	100	2
Canteen (Ramen)			
Beef	1/2 block	190	7
Cajun Chicken	1/2 block	190	7
Chicken	1/2 block	190	7
Chili	1/2 block	190	7
Hot & Spicy Vegetable	1/2 block	190	7
Texas Beef	1/2 block	190	7
Thai Chili Noodle	1 pack	780	12
Sugar, sweeteners, etc.			
Chow Hall			
Jelly – breakfast	1 ounce	100	4
Jelly – lunch	2 ounces	200	8
Sugar	2 packets	22	0
Syrup	3 ounces	200	0
Canteen			
Strawberry Spread	1 tablespoon	50	0
Sugar Cubes	1 cube	15	0
Sweet Sprinkles Sugar Substitute	1 packet	0	0
Busy Bee Honey	1 teaspoon	60	0
Vegetables			
Chow Hall			
Baked Potato	1 each	180	1
Beets	6 ounces	40	0
Blended Vegetables	6 ounces	40	0

Broccoli	6 ounces	40	0
Broccoli/Cauliflower	6 ounces	40	0
Cabbage Salad	6 ounces	115	0
Carrots	6 ounces	40	0
Chili Beans	4 ounces	120	1
Chopped Onions	1 serving	0	0
Corn	6 ounces	40	1
Cottage Fried Potatoes	6 ounces	240	1
French Fries	6 ounces	450	2
Fried Potatoes	6 ounces	210	3
Garlic Mashed Potatoes	6 ounces	140	6
Green Beans	6 ounces	40	0
Hash browns	6 ounces	150	1
Lettuce	11g serving	10	0
Mashed Potatoes	5 ounces	140	2
O'Brian Potatoes	6 ounces	150	1
Onions	1 ounce	0	0
Onions & Bell Peppers	2 ounces	90	0
Onions & Lettuce	1 serving	0	0
Onions & Pickles	1 serving	0	0
Parsley Carrots	5 ounces	40	0
Peas	6 ounces	90	0
Peas & Carrots	5 ounces	60	0
Pickles	1 serving	0	0
Pickles	4 each	0	0
Potatoes O'Brian	6 ounces	240	1
Potato Wedges - Baked	6 ounces	200	1
Refried Beans	6 ounces	165	3
Sauerkraut	2 ounces	10	0
Savory Style Beans	10 ounces	300	3
Seasoned Beans	4 ounces	120	1

Weight Loss Unlocked

Seasoned Beans	6 ounces	180	2
Seasoned Black Beans	5 ounces	180	2
Shredded Lettuce	1 serving	0	0
Spinach	5 ounces	40	0
Stir Fry Vegetables	6 ounces	60	0
Tatar Tots	6 ounces	350	1
Wax Beans	5 ounces	40	1
Zucchini	6 ounces	40	0
Canteen			
Hot Pickle	1 ounce	0	0
Kosher Pickle	1 ounce	0	0
Refried Beans	4 ounces	170	2

Six-ounce salad-veggie tray of the day (any vegetable or fruit salad) – no meat or cheese – 80-225 calories, 2 grams protein.

One bowl of green salad or cabbage wedge – 10-20 calories, 2 grams of carbs.

One-ounce salad dressing (depending on type, regular or lite) – 60-120 calories, 2 grams of carbs.

Eight-ounce steamed rice (white or brown) or 1 baked potato – 3 grams of protein, 200-220 calories.

Eight-ounce boiled beans (pinto, kidney, red or white) – 14 grams of protein, 200-250 calories.

Eight-ounce vegetables (cooked) – 5-6 grams of protein, 50-100 calories.

One serving (5 ounces) carrots, celery, turnips, radishes, broccoli, cauliflower, green onions, or cherry tomatoes – 1 gram of protein, approximately 50 calories.

One serving of bread of the day (2 slices of bread, 2 dinner rolls, 2 biscuits, 2 breadsticks, 2 tortillas, or 1 French bread, 1 bun, 1 serving cornbread) – 150-300 calories, 15-28 grams of carbs per each piece, 5-8 grams of protein.

A half ounce of margarine (whipped) – 90 calories, 10 grams of fat.

One serving of fresh fruit (apples, oranges, bananas or other seasonal fruit) – 60-120 calories, 24 grams of carbs.

Weight Loss Unlocked

Paul J.R. Dawson

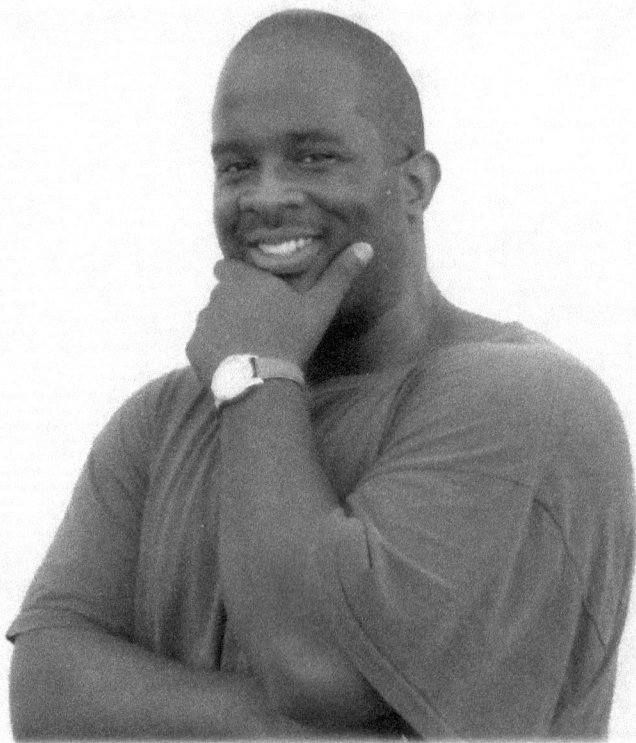

About the Author

Paul J.R. Dawson is an Oregon state inmate who is dedicating himself to revamping the prison industry from within through health, communication and financial freedom. His ultimate goal is to reduce recidivism by empowering those in custody to think outside the walls of prison. Mr. Dawson is currently a student at a Division I University and has a second book being published.

Coming 2021
Prisoner's Communication: Guidelines to Existing in Prison

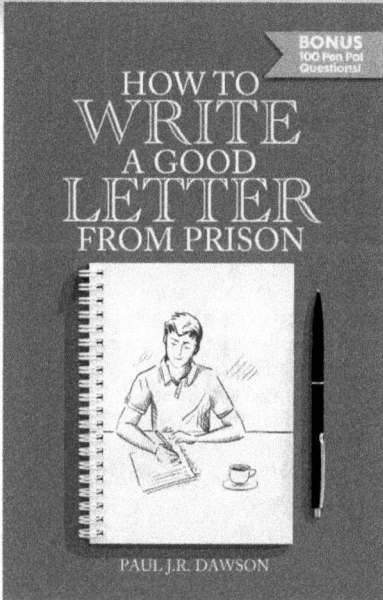

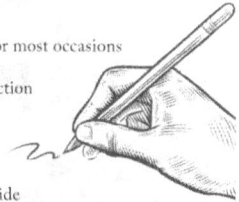

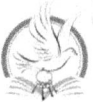

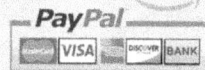

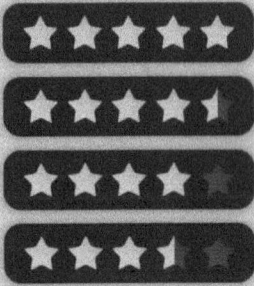

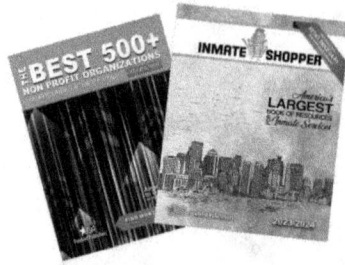

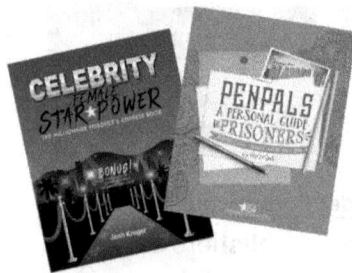

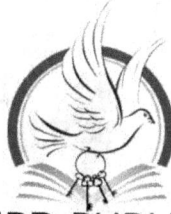

FREEBIRD PUBLISHERS

Thanks for your interest in Freebird Publishers!

We value our customers and would love to hear from you! Reviews are an important part in bringing you quality publications. We love hearing from our readers-rather it's good or bad (though we strive for the best)!

If you could take the time to review/rate any publication you've purchased with Freebird Publishers we would appreciate it!

If your loved one uses Amazon, have them post your review on the books you've read. This will help us tremendously, in providing future publications that are even more useful to our readers and growing our business.

Amazon works off of a 5 star rating system. When having your loved one rate us be sure to give them your chosen star number as well as a written review. Though written reviews aren't required, we truly appreciate hearing from you.

Sample Review Received on Inmate Shopper

poeticsunshine

★★★★★ **Truly a guide**

Reviewed in the United States on June 29, 2023

Verified Purchase

This book is a powerhouse of information. My son had to calm/ground himself to prioritize where to start.

Paul J.R. Dawson

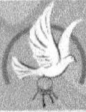

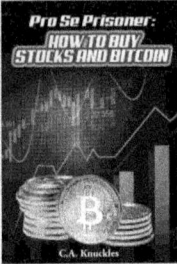

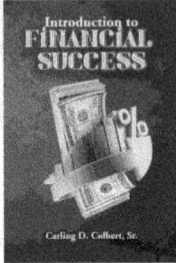

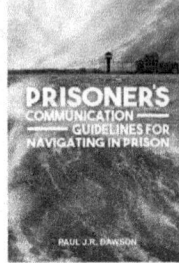

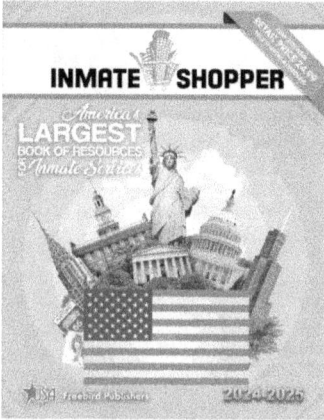

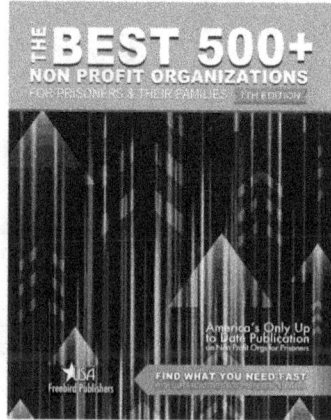

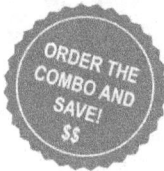

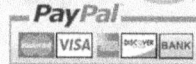

251

Paul J.R. Dawson

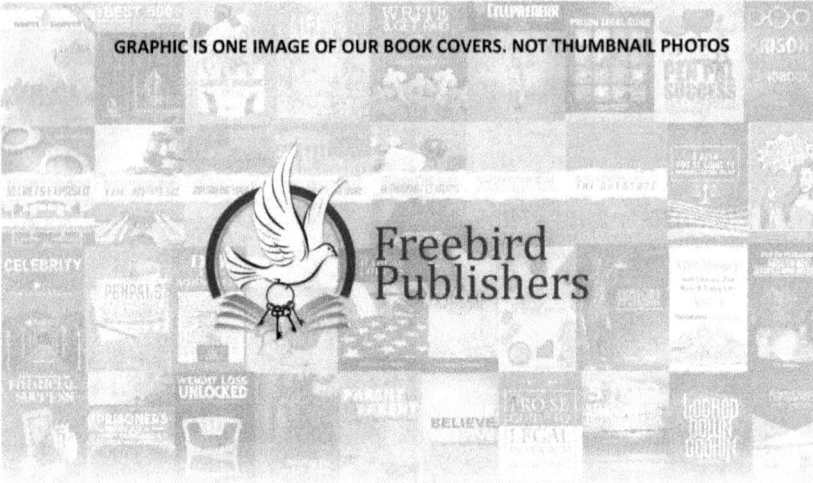

www.ingramcontent.com/pod-product-compliance
Lightning Source LLC
Chambersburg PA
CBHW070810270326
41927CB00010B/2369